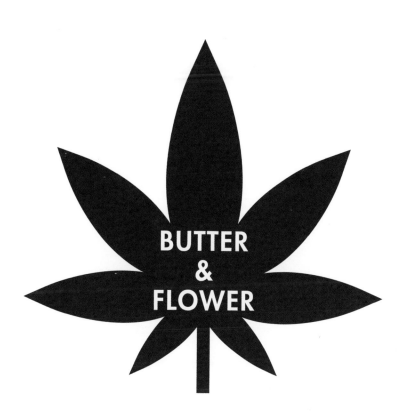

BUTTER & FLOWER

CANNABIS-INFUSED RECIPES AND STORIES FOR THE CANNACURIOUS

ANN ALLCHIN

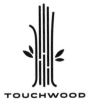

TOUCHWOOD

To my family, especially my parents,
who chose to approach the stigma of this
subject with encouragement.
(My kids, Reid and Charly, still eye-roll,
but they'll get over it.)

And to Kathie.

If we could see the miracle of a single flower clearly,
our whole life would change.

– Jack Kornfield, *Buddha's Little Instruction Book*

CONTENTS

STORIES

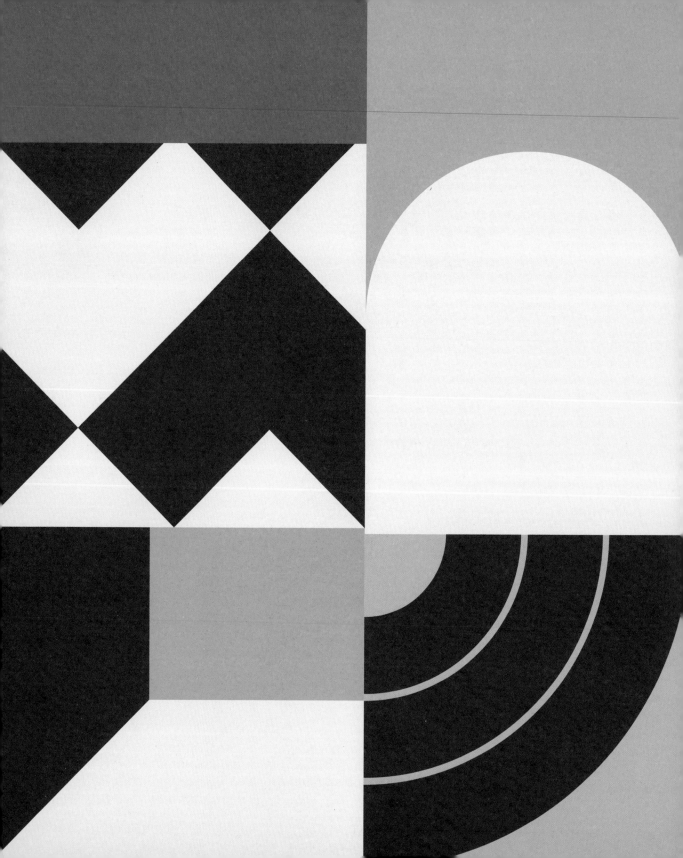

Introduction

My first joint was a lopsided thing that my friend Karen "rolled," with lined paper and masking tape. It was late at night in my second year of university, and I was visiting her in Montréal, somewhere in the neighbourhood of 1994 or '95. We didn't have papers, but I insisted on giving the devil's lettuce a try. Karen lit the thing and nearly set my face on fire. You would think a person would know intuitively how to inhale, but it appeared my lungs were more afraid of this new experience than I was. Let's blame Karen's joint.

Within a few months, though, I had figured things out. I toke, toke passed, and I was high! My mouth felt furry, and I appropriately stared off into space. I soon became a dabbler (not to be confused with a dabber—I'm still a bit of a lightweight).

At that time, I knew absolutely nothing about cannabis, its history, and how the drug worked. All I knew was that weed helped me analyze Superbowl commercials and get a good night's sleep when I had the Sunday blues.

Fast forward to about five (ten?) years ago, when my father-in-law's partner, Kathie, wasn't able to join us at our cottage due to yet another migraine. When Kathie isn't well, she's in bed for days at a time, crawling back and forth to the bathroom to be sick.

She's tried heavy prescription drugs, gluten-, dairy-, and sugar-free diets . . . she's even considered having her nerve endings burned off.

We figured that seeing whether cannabis might help was the least we could do.

Weed was still illegal in those days, but we ventured to a dark alley (ha!) and managed to find some. I started reading, baking, and sharing my creations. Yes, there was an incident where at a party, a drunk guy ate five brownies, went missing for a while, and ended up miming to a cab driver that he was lost and desperately needed to find his friend's couch. (They found him and tucked him in.) But when used as directed, the feedback I got on my edibles was very positive; they tasted great, the dosing was mild, and friends found the relief or relaxation they were looking for.

And Kathie? The damn headaches still get her. But she's a regular user of cannabis in different forms now, because since the first day she tried it, it's helped with the vomiting and her escape into sleep. Edibles still work best for her because they last the longest.

And as for me?

I truly never could have predicted that taking that first batch of infused chocolate chip cookies out of the oven would have led to where I am today. Baking and writing about cannabis brings so many elements of my person into one place.

I respect the truth of it—I like arguing with people who are misguided about its stigma, which was *politically intentional*. The history of cannabis is a social justice story, where the rights of the underrepresented, minorities, and the counterculture need to be protected. I want to fight for those rights, and telling cannabis stories is part of how I can do that.

I like the mischief of weed, the fun of bringing a tray of something delicious to a party, and helping people experiment with something new (yet harmless). And obviously, I like spending time in the kitchen. Don't tell my husband this when I'm tired and feel like going out, though.

I like helping people, and gifting. The medicinal element of cannabis is an easy one. The fact that sick people are still denied access to something natural that can help with pain, and that is under-researched for so many other conditions . . . Let's just say that it pains me (sorry) that sharing edibles is still so hard in so many places. Oh, and PS, I have a neuroscience degree! Who knew that that damn piece of paper would ever become relevant? But when I started reading about the endocannabinoid system and how much of the science supported the medicinal cannabis claims, I was sold on becoming an advocate.

And recreationally? I'm very live and let live. You do you. Unless you're too young, are pregnant, or are operating some kind of vehicle, and then watch my hammer come down. Be smart. That's another thing about me—I'm happy to have a wee cannaplatform, as I will always be a voice for safety.

I also encourage casual cannabis use. You don't need to be an extreme recreational user to enjoy a little pot. Try one of my recipes and share it with friends, just "start low and go slow." (That phrase is so common for edibles that I don't think I even have to pay someone to quote it. Imagine.) Cannabis is much more individual than drinking. Listen to your own body, experiment a little, and learn about what might work for you. I happen to be more of a "solo smoker" so that I don't get too introverted at parties, and that's okay! Like I said, you do you.

Finally, I'm proud that I've been able to use my skills as an editor and listener to share the cannabis interviews within this book. I feel honoured to have spoken with such incredible people who have had transformative relationships with this natural plant. The more stories we're able to share, the more comfortable society will be with exploring and researching choices and natural healing options.

A sincere thank you to everyone who shared their stories within these pages. I'm so pleased to have met you.

I'm looking forward to connecting with you, my dear reader, to talk more about this incredible plant and your own experiences. I hope you enjoy my fun take on what has been a life-changing experience for so many.

ABOUT THIS BOOK

Obviously, this book is about to be the coolest one on your shelf. Here's how to use it.

Start by reading the following section, Safety and Health. This is mandatory.

Browse through the other sections in this introduction. I've done the math for you regarding dosing as long as you monkey see, monkey do how I calculate my infusions and treats—check out the foundational recipes and the dosing for each creation to see how this works. I've found that most who enjoy edibles like a lower dose. (You can always eat more.) If, however, you're like most of my Instagram followers and have a high tolerance for weed, you're going to have to make modifications to my assumptions; there's advice for this in the math section.

My recipes are very "stay in your lane," straightforward baking. Making infused butter, oil, alcohol, or sugar is a little time consuming, so I didn't want to add to that with complex recipes. Plus, failures are much more expensive with edibles! I also believe that edibles should be measurable by piece, for the most part, so that dosing doesn't get confusing,

and that the remainder of a batch should be able to be frozen so that treats can be enjoyed over time. Hence (yes, I just said "hence," I'm basically a knight of the round table), you'll see a lot of delicious cookies in these pages.

And hey, I spoke with some incredible people for this book! Go ahead and take a break from the kitchen to read an inspirational story about a transformational history with cannabis. If you've even cracked the cover, you likely have an open mind, but you might be surprised by what you learn, or by how your heart feels, at the end of one of these stories. I'll probably get in sh&t from my editor for how long these pieces are, but I'm a reader, and am confident that there are still others like me out there who are not just TikToking . . . Wait a minute, TikToking? Now there's an app I can get behind!

Anyway, I wouldn't be surprised if these stories turned you from a toke dipper to an activist. If so, my work here is done.

SAFETY AND HEALTH

Here are the rules:

1. Start low and go slow.
Wow, it's only been a few pages, and I've already said this twice. I must mean it.

Edibles are different from smoking. They take longer to kick in, and they stay in your system for longer, sometimes up to twelve hours. Plan ahead and don't drive during this time.

Dosing for a novice cannabis user is usually 5 to 10 mg THC per piece.

Don't get impatient, thinking you can't feel the edible, and eat more. This is a common mistake that sometimes results in regrets. After you try a treat, it can take an hour to an hour and a half to kick in, and sometimes even longer on a full stomach. Learn about your tolerance and your body with small doses—start with half a treat. You can always eat more later.

No one has ever overdosed on pot, but plenty have had anxiety attacks. If you're feeling "greened out," rest in a quiet place among loved ones, and if you're truly concerned, get medical help.

Go ahead and message me if you want more advice, or if I can help with your comfort level. Or just if you're bored and lonely: annallchin.com.

2. Label edibles to avoid accidental ingestion.
I had super cool stickers made, and I know you want to be me. But a permanent marker will also do the trick. No surprises.

3. Don't drive, operate machinery, or go to work after indulging.
Some old-school cannabis smokers seem to think they can drive post weed. I blame prohibition and lack of

PR for this. When you're not fully on your game for any reason, don't drive.

Maybe if you're a rock star, I'll support you going to work on my edibles. Or maybe if you work at a grow op. Okay, it appears there are some exceptions to this rule, but for the most part? Save the cookies for when you're not punching a time card.

4. Don't mix.
Again, some exceptions: Charlie Sheen. Miley Cyrus. Keith Richards. You? Don't walk and chew gum at the same time.

5. Be a good parent to children and pets.
I encourage conversations with kids rather than hiding cookies. Those little minxes could find them, and because I created these recipes, I know they're delicious. There's no reason to be ashamed of cannabis use anymore, so educate your kids with a clear "don't touch" policy.

When my kids were little I would lock edibles in a cash bag in the freezer. Teens will find those keys, so you're going to have to be even more creative. Be as good a parent as you are on your best day. The same goes for pets. (Only the really smart cats will find those keys.) Ask an open-minded, qualified vet if looking to medicate an animal in pain, but otherise, keep all treats well out of reach.

6. If you have health conditions or questions, consult a doctor.
The medical community is finally becoming more informed on the ganja. If your doctor is an anti-weedosaurus and you think that cannabis might be able to help with your condition, go ahead and hunt for a new one. But do get medical advice—I'm

surprisingly skilled with a pair of tweezers and a sliver, but regrettably, I am not a doctor. If you have a family history of mental health or substance abuse conditions, medical advice is even more important.

With pregnancy, again, ask your doctor. Cannabis does have an affinity for fats, and it does accumulate in breast milk. Personally, I kept my pregnancies substance-free, but I know that through history, cannabis has been useful in labour. Ask your doctor.

7. Consent

Slipping someone a special cookie might have made for a funny *Three's Company* episode, but it's not funny in real life. Eyes wide open. Offer politely, and respect boundaries.

8. Legalities, including travel

Observe the laws where you live, and don't cross borders with cannabis, even if it's legal in both places—that's still trafficking (although you can travel with it within Canada, eh?!). But don't end up a drug mule. Read Audrey's story (page 70) in this book for a cautionary tale.

9. Youth

Observe the legal age for THC indulgence where you live. There have been questions about how a developing endocannabinoid system might be affected by cannabis, how earlier use might lead to more chronic use, and how predisposed mental health conditions might present earlier with use. It's probably best to wait to try it until your brain cells start dying off like mine have, unless there's a health condition that could benefit from cannabis medication, in which case, see that "consult a doctor" advice, above.

***

Now that I've done the dirty work with my words of caution about cannabis use, let's go ahead and celebrate the medicinal goodness it can bring! I partly became an advocate for this plant because its properties are shockingly counterintuitive. Anything that feels good is not good for you, too, right? Wrong! Weed can be enjoyable, relaxing, and…

Note that these are cherry-picked single research papers of evidence (see Notes on page 230 for all of the nitty gritty). I tried to find review papers, which are scientists giving broad opinions based on a bunch of studies. Yes, this is sparse, but this is a cookbook, not a nerd party. At the same time, I want you to know that cannabis claims are not just pothead hearsay.

* Cannabis is not a gateway drug.[1]
* A good way to understand drug risk is through the "Margin of Exposure," which is a ratio of the toxicity of a drug and how much people take of it. Coles notes: a high score is a good thing. Alcohol, nicotine, cocaine, and heroin fall into the high risk category with MOEs less than 10. Cannabis is considered low risk, with an MOE greater than 10,000.[2] Plus, I'm pretty sure it's never killed any lab bunnies, even if you get them super stoned. No humans, either.
* Although it's most healthy with all elements of the plant working together (this is the "entourage effect," and what is meant when you see "full spectrum" on a cannabis product),[3] properties can be modified to reduce psychoactivity.
* You can enjoy cannabis medicine entirely under your own oversight, from seed to use

* There's evidence that some cannabis properties may prevent cancers,[4] and can ease cancer symptoms, including loss of appetite, anxiety, nausea,[5] and pain.[6]
* Cannabis is anti-inflammatory, antioxidant, antimicrobial, and analgesic (pain killing).[6,4]
* CBD might help with memory[7] and shows promise for the treatment and prevention of Alzheimer's disease.[8]
* Cannabis can prevent convulsions and treat epilepsy.[9]
* Cannabis can help with anxiety[4] (although as we know, it can also exacerbate anxiety; get help from an experienced budtender, and experiment in a mentally safe space).
* CBD has been found to be useful in the treatment of diseases and conditions associated with inflammation, such as Crohn's disease, ulcerative colitis, Parkinson's disease, atopic dermatitis, and psoriasis.[10]
* Cannabis can help with many of our regulation-related conditions, like menopause,[11] sleep, and hunger. (I'm not exercising my internet finger to find refs on sleep and hunger; it's just recognized as a fact by now that cannabis helps to treat insomnia and can stimulate appetite for sick people.
* CBD helps with migraine relief.[12] (The study I referenced reports reduction in headache and migraine severity by 50 percent.)
* Cannabis can relieve eye pressure, helping with glaucoma. There's truth in the jest that someone is "treating their glaucoma." It's short-term and can lend itself to other complications, though.[13]
* Cannabis can serve as an effective substitute for other drugs.[14,15] (Hey, the author of one of the papers I referenced, Philippe Lucas, is the same Philippe Lucas who Sarah Campbell mentions in her story, page 39! Small world.)
* Weed can fight herpes replication. That's right, I said herpes. The evidence was just a petri dish study from 1980, but I wasn't about to miss the opportunity to say "herpes" in a cookbook.[16]
* Cannabis is a neuroprotectant, having been patented by the U.S. government as one in 1998, despite still being classified a Schedule I drug at time of writing.

Other concerns? Here's what I know. (Reminder: Not a doctor. But I do dabble in science for my other job as a medical writer.)

* About 9 percent of cannabis users have symptoms of dependence.[17] Markers of addiction are present with cannabis, but "may not be as robust as other drugs of abuse."[18] However, no one is selling their house to pay for their ever-increasing cannabis habit (reference: Ann Allchin, cannabaker extraordinaire).
* Cannabis withdrawal symptoms include irritability, anger or aggression, anxiety, sleep difficulty, decreased appetite, restlessness, depressed mood, shakiness, overheating, chills, and headaches.[19] But since I'm a pot baker and not a real scientist, I'll add that I think this only happens after withdrawal from chronic use, and that it passes within a few weeks.
* Long-term effects on IQ, learning, and memory seem inconclusive, but starting young doesn't help.[18]
* Memory and learning, attention, and psychomotor ability have been found to be less impaired in regular versus non-regular cannabis

users. In other words, potheads can build some tolerance to being impaired. Tolerance may strike some as a positive at first—look, heavier users can function better!—but it also means that extreme recreational users will hunt for more intense cannabis experiences, which is not necessarily a positive.[20]

* There's been talk of cannabis aggravating schizophrenia. There has been no evidence that cannabis causes schizophrenia, but it might not do the symptoms any favours. Cannabis use is on the rise, but the rate of schizophrenia has not increased.[21]

This list is in no way exhaustive, and luckily, now that public cannabis policy is finally opening up, new research is constantly bringing science-based revelations to light. Run away (Monty Python? Anyone?) and do your own research. I can guarantee that as a cannaphile, you'll like much of what you see.

WHAT TO KNOW WHEN BUYING CANNABIS

As MC Hammer would say, let's break it down:

* More than 100 cannabinoids have been identified in weed, and the more your body has access to, the better it is for your health. (This is "the entourage effect," that I mentioned earlier.) THC and CBD are the two most well-known cannabinoids; THC is your buzz-o-meter, while CBD is good for general health and contrasts the buzz of THC (CBD can also be taken alone like a non-psychoactive multivitamin). High THC and low CBD will give the greatest stoned results, if that's what you're going for. Balance between the two cannabinoids will reduce the high and work well medicinally.

* Decide whether you're looking for an energetic (sativa) or relaxed (indica) feeling. Sativas and indicas were once distinct species of cannabis, but most strains available today are a hybrid of the two. In truth, descriptors with X/X percent sativa/indica usually apply more to connoisseurs' assessments of a strain's impact rather than actual lab-tested scientific breakdowns. Browse indica/sativa blends and reviews of cultivars until you find one available to you that sounds about right for the effects you're trying to achieve.

* Check your purse or murse (Cheers, Seinfeld), and decide how much you want to spend. I'd recommend at least infusing a block of butter (2 cups or 454 g) or the equivalent with 7 g (¼ oz) of cannabis bud, and that concentration is what estimates in this book are based on.

* Terpenes are further compounds in cannabis and other plants that change the taste of a cannabis strain. With edibles, taste will be overwhelmed by other ingredients, but terpenes also tweak the effects of a strain. For example, limonene in cannabis (also found in lemons!) may reduce anxiety, while pinene in cannabis (also found in pine trees!) may help with pain relief. When you've narrowed down the other aspects of a cultivar, browse the terpene profiles. Those effects might just give one strain edge over another for you at time of purchase, and if you're going to smoke any of what you've chosen, terpene blends will be more important for flavour/smell.

* Make the final call by going for the cutest strain name. *Crouching Tiger Hidden Alien*? I'd probably go for that one without reading anything else.

KEY CANNATERMS

Weed has a lot of industry-specific lingo. Here's a list that I hope isn't too general or too specialized that can be a gateway (ha ha) to whatever you're looking to learn. I've included the concentrates terms also, but if you're more of a lightweight (like me), I'd suggest sticking with your cookies. As an edibles cookbook author, though, I might just be biased!

Term	Definition
420	It's thought that 420 started among a group of friends in California in the seventies called the Waldos, who met to smoke weed regularly at 4:20 PM. Now, 420 (April 20) has become a day to celebrate all things cannabis.
bhang	A cannabis drink with a long history in India.
BHO	Butane hash oil, the most common extraction method used to create concentrates. Don't try this at home.
budtender	Your weed helper at a dispensary.
cannabinoids	The compounds of the cannabis plant.
CBD	One of the two most famous cannabinoids. CBD is responsible for many of the medicinal properties of cannabis, and it counteracts the high of THC. CBD is not psychoactive when taken alone; many take it for health benefits in a similar way to a multivitamin.
clone	A cutting from another cannabis plant that grows into its own plant. Clones are a good way to avoid growing plants from seed.
cola	The flowering part of a cannabis plant.
concentrates	The chemicals of cannabis without the plant matter. Concentrates have higher amounts of cannabinoids and terpenes than the plant itself. Extracts are types of concentrates that are created using solvents, but concentrates can also be made mechanically or physically. Concentrates can have 80 percent or more THC while regular herb has an average of 15 or 20 percent.

cultivar	Another word for strain. This is the type of cannabis bred for specific characteristics. Weed nerds like my canna-fact-checker, Jason, wish I would always say cultivar, but c'est la Dutchie.
dab/dabbing	Heating a (strong) concentrate to a potent vapour that can be inhaled. This takes a fancy rig that I don't know how to use because I'm a lightweight. Terpenes and flavonoids are maintained here, though, so the individual taste and character of a strain can be truly appreciated.
decarboxylation	The process of removing an acid molecule from naturally occurring THCA/ CBDA using heat to get THC/CBD, which are more useful by the body's receptors for therapeutic effects. The lighter or heat source automatically does this with smoking, but for edibles, additional heat is required ahead of time to achieve the expected effects of THC/CBD.
endocannabinoids and the endocannabinoid system	Discovered in 1992 by Dr. Raphael Mechoulam and his team, the endocannabinoid system (ECS) is our internal system of regulation; endocannabinoids are home-grown neurotransmitters acting throughout the body, managing regulatory functions like healing, appetite, memory, mood, pain, sleep, and thermoregulation. Cannabinoids are external chemicals that stand in for endocannabinoids, affecting the ECS in various ways.
extracts	A subgroup of concentrates that use solvents to create high cannabinoid and terpene substances from the cannabis plant.
fan leaves	The big iconic leaves of the cannabis plant. Fan leaves are low in cannabinoids.
feminized	Only female cannabis plants flower, which is where the beloved cannabinoids are (girl power). If male plants are prevented from pollinating female plants, the resin is more plentiful and full of the desired cannabinoids. "Feminized" seeds can be purchased that only carry female genes, thereby avoiding the risk of getting male plants from seed.
flavonoids	Nearly every plant has flavonoids; they're responsible for variation in colour, flavour, aroma, nutrition, and health. There are twenty flavonoids among varieties of cannabis, adding flavour/scent/appearance variation and (possibly) nutrition and health, in addition to those offered by differences in cannabinoids and terpenes.

flower	Synonymous with "bud." The bloom of the female cannabis plant where the useful compounds are concentrated.
ghee	Clarified butter, with milk solids removed, popular in India. Some believe that ghee improves potency of cannabis infusions. Ghee has a higher smoke point than butter, so it's sometimes preferable to use over butter when cooking with high heat.
hash	A cannabis concentrate made by mechanically removing resin from cannabis and compacting it into a block.
hemp	The non-intoxicating varieties of the *Cannabis*[22] plant (containing less than 0.3 percent THC). CBD can be extracted from hemp or THC-rich cannabis, but hemp has more CBD available and can help avoid legal complications.
hybrid	A cross between indica and sativa strains. Most modern strains are hybrids due to a long history of cross-breeding.
ice water hash/ bubble hash	A concentrate made by freezing trichomes and separating them from the plant using ice water and mesh bags. People dab it (or sprinkle it onto a joint).
indica	Traditionally, indicas were a short, stocky species of cannabis plants with wide leaves that grew fine in cold climates. Now, due to advancements in cultivation methods, although physical traits are still useful for differentiation, indica refers more to the effects of the strain; indica-dominant cultivars often give a more relaxed, sleepy feeling.
kief	Resin glands that fall from the buds to the bottom of your grinder or jar, or when sifted through a screen.
kush	A lineage of cannabis cultivars most likely originating from the popular OG Kush.
landrace	Original Darwinian-style strains that developed in the wild, without human intervention. Today, all strains can be traced back to their landraces and they often carry the names of the terroir where they originated (e.g., *Thai, Hindu Kush, Acapulco Gold*).

marijuana	Term for cannabis popularized in the 1930s to tie xenophobia and racism toward Hispanics to drug use.
OG	"Ocean grown," as in coastal California, or "original gangster" out of the L.A. hip hop scene in the 80s/90s via Cypress Hill, or for the term "overgrow the government," or "original growers," or just "original." With cannabis, OG usually refers to some kind of lineage related to OG Kush.
pistils	Wispy white hairs and their ovaries on the cannabis plant trying to capture pollen. Pistils turn orange, red, or brown closer to harvest time. A grower makes sure the pistils don't trap pollen if he or she is going for sensimilla (see definition below). The longer a pistil is sexually frustrated, the more resin it develops to trap pollen. We like resin.
psychoactive	Mind-altering.
resin	The sappy substance on the trichomes of cannabis flowers containing the highest concentration of cannabinoids.
sativa	Traditionally, sativas were tall, spidery-leafed plants that liked warm climates. Now, due to advancements in cultivation methods, although physical traits are still useful for differentiation, sativa refers more to the effects of the strain; sativa-dominant cultivars often give a more energetic, productive feeling.
Schedule I	At time of writing, cannabis is still considered a Schedule I drug in the U.S. (I suspect and hope that this will change soon and age my book.) Schedule I is defined as having no medicinal value and high potential for abuse. Other Schedule I drugs include LSD and heroin.
sensimilla	Means seedless. Unfertilized cannabis plants generally produce more resin, and therefore more cannabinoids, improving potency.
strain	The type of cannabis bred for specific characteristics (e.g., *Chocolope, Sour Diesel, OG Kush Breath*).
sugar leaves	The little leaves closest to the flowers. These get "trimmed" off because they're not great to smoke, but they still have high resin and cannabinoids, so they can be a good (and cheap) option for baking.

terpenes	Chemical compounds found in plants, including cannabis. Terpenes add differentiation in flavour, smell, and (possibly) effects between strains.
THCA, THC	The main psychoactive compound in cannabis. THCA is the acid precursor to THC, present in the natural plant.
tincture	An alcohol- or glycerin-based cannabis liquid. Administration is usually sublingual (under the tongue) as it's quicker than swallowing and going through the digestive tract.
topicals	Cannabis-based lotions, balms, or oils used on the skin to treat mostly inflammation, pain, or skin conditions.
trichomes	The little microscopically mushroom-shaped glands that produce the resin on cannabis flowers. Colour change through the growth cycle can lead growers through the desired effects they want out of the plant. The trichomes are the powerhouse of the plant.
trim and shake	The bits of bud, trichomes, kief, and sugar leaves that are removed or fall off through cannabis processing. Trim is considered low-grade (and harsh) for smoking, so is used in hash or edibles, or is thrown out. Shake can be used for hash, edibles, or pre-rolls, but quality and strain can be variable. Both are cost effective.
vaping	What your fourteen-year-old is doing on the schoolyard with tobacco these days (ugh). Vaping cannabis happens at a lower temperature, avoiding traditional combustion. Odours tend to be more discreet, and it's assumed that some of the more dangerous side effects of combustion are avoided. Terpenes and other compounds that might burn off at higher temperatures are also more likely to be maintained.
wax, shatter, and more	Cannabis concentrates with CO_2, BHO, ethanol, or without a solvent, to be dabbed, sprinkled on flower, used with a dab rig, vaped with a wax pen . . . Probably too much for this lightweight over here. Maybe someday I'll try it. Maybe someday I'll bungee jump, but that's just about as likely.

MATH, ASSUMPTIONS, AND HOW TO READ THE RECIPES

I feel like I'm talking too much, so let's make this quick.

* Drool over a food photo in this book. Take note of what kind of infusion the recipe uses—cannabutter, cannacoconut oil, cannavirgin olive oil, cannasugar, or alcohol tincture (that last one is just for one recipe, Peach Gummies [see page 225], and you'll find the method within that recipe).

* Buy your weed, based on the section "What to Know When Buying Cannabis" (see page 15). Or maybe you grew your own or were gifted weed—good for you!

* Return to the original recipe you wanted to try. Take note of the dosing strength. *The dosing I've worked out should be okay for the average bear.* If you think this might be too strong for you, though, change some of the cannabutter out for regular butter (or oil or sugar, you get me). If you think the strength will be too weak, you have five options:

    1. Increase the concentration of THC in your weed to higher than 16 percent.
    2. Swap fat/sugar amounts in the recipe for more infused butter or oil. (Many of the recipes also use regular fats or sugars.)
    3. Increase the amount of cannabis you put into your cannabutter, coconut oil, olive oil, or sugar foundational recipe beyond what I suggest in that section.
    4. Eat more pieces.
    5. Some combination of the above.

* If you're playing with dosing strength, go ahead and use my friend Jeffthe420chef's dosing calculator (jeffthe420chef.com/calculator). It's great and will work out per-piece strengths.

* Prepare your infusion from the Foundational Recipes section (see page 25).

* Prepare the recipe. Just as a note: my difficulty levels and strain recommendations are all just for fun. All recipes are pretty easy, and depending on where you live, strains can be hard to come by. I just suggested relevant cultivars for each recipe to get you thinking about the growers and how creative they can be. Diversity is a beautiful thing.

TOOLKIT

Key Tools

* Kitchen scale—Look, before I was a pot baker I baked with measuring cups and spoons without weighing a damn thing, too. But you're going to need to weigh your infusions for each recipe and put the rest away for later. Scales are cheap. Remember to zero the scale with a bowl on it and then add the cannabis, butter, or oil.

* 1 Tbsp cookie dough scoop—Measuring properly is important for dosing consistency.

* Double boiler—A heat-proof bowl over a pot of simmering water also works well.

* Silicone baking mats or parchment paper

* Baking sheets

* Cheesecloth or a fine sieve

* Enticing Netflix programs and a kitchen TV

* 8 × 8 or 9 × 9–inch square pan for squares

* Rolling pin

- Cooking spray
- Candy thermometer
- Pastry brush
- Pizza cutter
- Cooling rack

Optional but Useful Tools

- I adore my stand mixer. You can get away with not having one, but it's the bomb. And it looks class on your counter.
- I also adore my food processor. I've broken about five of them. I don't recommend getting impatient and shoving a wooden spoon in.
- I like glass snap lid containers for infused butters and oils. They're better for pouring hot products into, to save for later.
- A slow cooker is great for infusions, and your grandma can probably lend you one.

Special Tools for Certain Recipes

- Cannabis leaf (buy online), snowflake, or other cool cookie cutters for cut outs
- Piping bags, tips, and colours for the decorative cookie recipes
- Squeeze bottles and funnels for decorating and gummies
- 8-inch round cake pan in case you'd like to make a wee Raspberry Chocolate Celebration Cake (see page 75). An offset spatula (icing spreader) and a pastry scraper (dough cutter) are helpful for the cake, too.
- 6 fluted tart pans with removable bottoms are needed for the Black Forest Cheesecake Tarts (see page 79).
- Hunt down some pretty mini muffin cups for the Mocha Hazelnut Truffles (see page 89).
- A silicone macaron mat helps to manage sizing for the Lime Passion Fruit Sandwich Cookies

(see page 95) and the Caramelized Onion Blue Cheese Not-Gougères (see page 211).
- Large flat spatulas are helpful to shift the flatbreads around (see page 215). Try the dollar/junk store.
- Cannabis leaf silicone candy moulds work well for the gummies (see page 225). You can find them online.
- Get a microplane. You're going to love me for that advice. (Plus, it will help with zesting lemons and grating Parm for a few recipes in this book.)
- If you want pizzelle (see page 131), there's no getting around having a pizzelle maker. I know it's coin, but you'll use it. Think pretty cookie gifting.
- You'll need a silicone cupcake pan or two for the Persian-Style Honey Saffron Brittle (see page 151).
- I love my squares pan. It's like a muffin pan but with squares. This will help with the Pecan Pie Squares (see page 157) and the Cranberry Wheaten Toasts (see page 205), and you can make brownies with it, too (see page 81).

In Case You're Wealthy

- Sous vide machines aren't too much coin, and supposedly they also contain the smell when making infusions (I haven't tried one personally).
- There are a number of futuristic infusion machines on the market that do a lot of the monitoring/timing work for you while containing the smell. But they're *money*, as they'd say in *Swingers*. So I've never tried the fancy ones. Because they're *money*.

ABOUT THE STORIES

I thoroughly enjoyed interviewing everyone I spoke with for this book. I was introduced to some people through friends; with others, I just found something interesting in their Instagram profiles and suggested a blind phone "date." I made a conscious effort to present diverse perspectives on all things cannabis. I only had to give one person I approached the "it's not you, it's me" break-up conversation prior to an interview. Can you believe my luck?

A few things to note: my process was to have an informal conversation with each person, following his or her lead and asking more about what I found interesting. I recorded our conversation, skittered away, typed the entire chat out, and then edited our talk for length, order of events, to (mostly) remove myself, and to make it stronger on the written page. Many of the interviewees might have written more beautiful prose if left to themselves, but I liked the cooperative and casual nature of our discussions. After I was through cutting and pasting, everyone edited further to their own satisfaction.

I'm really very proud of the perspectives participants had the bravery to share.

The last thing I want to sound like is a lawyer, but I will say that many of our interview relationships were new, so although we agree regarding most things weed, there's a chance we might disagree on many other things, and that participants might disagree with one another; hence, "the opinions expressed in these stories represent the views of the speakers and do not necessarily reflect the views of me, the other participants, or anyone other than themselves," blah blah blah. Is the draft dodger from the Shuswap happy that his story is in the same book as the octogenarian drug mule from Calgary? The truth is that I suspect they'd get along, but I didn't give them the opportunity to get to know each other and decide, and I did not spend days scouring social media accounts for anything that might feed cancel culture. Because I care, but I don't care. I respect that we might not agree on soup to nuts, although I like both soup and nuts.

So. Take the stories as they are, which is beautiful and heartfelt, in my humble opinion. And the rest? Keep an open mind and an open heart.

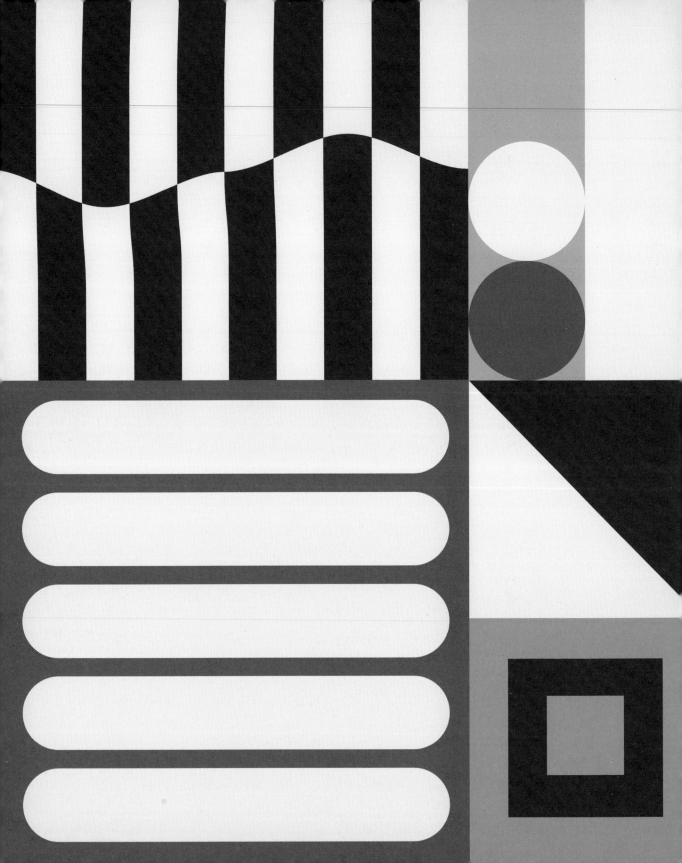

FOUNDATIONAL RECIPES

Cannabutter, Cannacoconut Oil, and CannaVirgin Olive Oil

While the stovetop method is the quickest and most accessible way to make cannabutter or oil, unfortunately, it will also make your house smell like a skunk brothel. You may want to wait to make infusions until you know your mother-in-law or the tax auditor isn't due for a visit. You can use a slow cooker and leave your infusion untended for longer, but if you make edibles regularly, consider investing in a hands-off appliance that also contains the smell (ask a budtender for advice).

BAG OF TRICKS

Kitchen scale

Double boiler (or medium saucepan with heat-proof bowl), or slow cooker

Candy thermometer (optional)

Cheesecloth or fine sieve

Sunflower lecithin (optional—can be purchased in health food stores or online)

DOSE ASSUMPTIONS

Here we're performing an extraction with 7 g (¼ oz) of decarboxylated cannabis bud containing about 16 percent THC and 2 cups (454 g) unsalted butter, which should yield about 18 mg THC per Tbsp.

If using 454 g of coconut oil or 2 cups of cannavirgin olive oil, yields will be a little lower, at about 11 mg THC per Tbsp.

TIMING

1 hour for decarboxylation

3 hours for simmering (or 8–12 hours in a slow cooker)

10 minutes for sieving and fussing about

1 hour in the fridge to allow the butter/coconut oil to resolidify for removal of water

INGREDIENTS

7 g (¼ oz) cannabis bud at approximately 16 percent THC content. (Don't stress too much about finding this percentage. Bodily effects don't shift greatly with minimal variation here.)

2 cups (454 g) unsalted butter, coconut oil that's solid at room temperature, or extra-virgin olive oil

1 Tbsp sunflower lecithin (optional—helps with overall consistency)

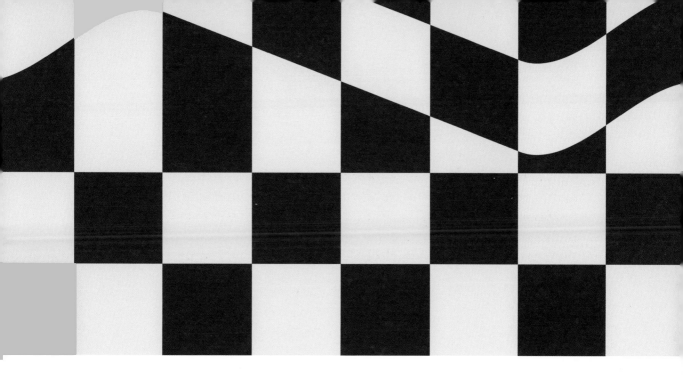

Decarboxylate your cannabis by baking it in an oven-safe dish at 240°F for 1 hour. (This "activates" the THC and CBD by converting them from their acid forms.)

Add about 2 inches of water to a medium saucepan, bring to a moderate boil, and set a heat-proof bowl on top, or use a double boiler, which is less likely to tip. Add 2 cups of butter and the lecithin (optional) to the bowl and allow it to melt. (I'm just going to call it butter from here on in—substitute in your mind for coconut or olive oils as needed.) Add 1 cup of water (with butter only) and your bud. (Or add water, butter, and bud to slow cooker. Skip adding water if infusing olive oil, as you won't be able to separate it later. But be sure to keep temperatures low.)

Allow the butter to heat without boiling for 3 hours (if you have a candy thermometer, aim for 160–200°F), stirring occasionally and making sure the saucepan doesn't boil dry. (Or cook using a low-heat setting for 8–12 hours in a slow cooker.) This process extracts the THC from the green and binds it to the butter.

Congrats, you now have cannabutter! Allow the magic you've created to cool until you can comfortably work with it, but make sure it stays liquid.

Pour the cannabutter through a cheesecloth or fine sieve into a container. (Take care not to use plastic if the butter is still too warm.) Press as much butter out of the cheesecloth as you can, and discard the now-useless plant matter.

Chill the cannabutter in the fridge. When solid, lift the infused butter from the container and turf the water that has separated to the bottom. Label and store the cannabutter in the fridge or freezer for later use—I usually go for freezing it because it's heartbreaking to toss a precious infusion over concerns it's gone bad. Don't reheat cannabutter in the microwave.

Cannasugar

While binding THC to fats is the more traditional way to bake with pot, some recipes offer more play if sugars are used instead. Making edibles using this method greatly decreases the stink factor; however, there is the potential for more variability in dosing due to potential differences in alcohol strength, rest time, and agitation.

BAG OF TRICKS

Mason jar

Plastic gloves

Cheesecloth or fine sieve

Baking sheet lined with parchment paper
   or a silicone baking mat

Food processor

DOSE ASSUMPTIONS

Here we're performing an extraction with 7 g (¼ oz) of decarboxylated cannabis bud containing 16 percent THC (don't stress about the percentage; if there is a variation, it should be all good), ½ cup (120 mL) of the highest proof alcohol your local liquor store offers (I think we're regulated to 40 percent here because it's all I could find, but feel free to go higher if you can), and 1 cup of sugar. Using this combo, we can assume that each Tbsp of cannasugar contains about 3 mg THC.

TIMING

1 hour for decarboxylation

45 minutes to a few days to let the cannabis
   infuse with the alcohol

10 minutes for sieving, fussing about, adding
   sugar to alcohol, and spreading sugar
   mixture across the baking sheet

At least 1 hour to bake the sugar dry

5 minutes to process the sugar

INGREDIENTS

7 g (¼ oz) cannabis

½ cup (120 mL) highest proof alcohol available

1 cup sugar

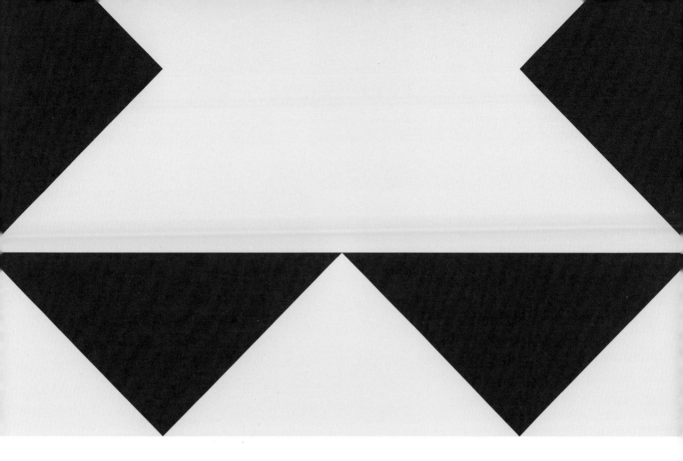

Decarboxylate your cannabis. (Bake in Pyrex dish at 240°F for 1 hour.)

Add weed to a small jar with a lid and pour in the alcohol (a large jar won't submerge the bud). Secure the lid and leave the jar on the counter, shaking it occasionally, for a minimum of 45 minutes. Adding time to this process will darken the colour and improve results.

Put on gloves—the alcohol may transfer some THC to you through your fingertips; maybe my love of pot has just made me paranoid, but if you have plans later, better safe than sorry. Strain the liquid through the cheesecloth or sieve into a bowl and press out as much alcohol as possible. Discard the plant matter.

Add the sugar to the canna-alcohol.

Preheat the oven to 250°F. Spread the sugar mixture evenly across the baking sheet and bake for 1 hour, stirring a few times, until the sugar becomes golden and dry. When you remove the baking sheet to stir the sugar, try not to breathe in, unless you want to do Polish wedding receiving-line shots with your lungs (which you might, who am I to judge).

When finished, the cannasugar should be quite crisp. Carefully put it in a food processor and pulse to a powder.

Store your herbal, sugary sweetness in a dry place until ready for use.

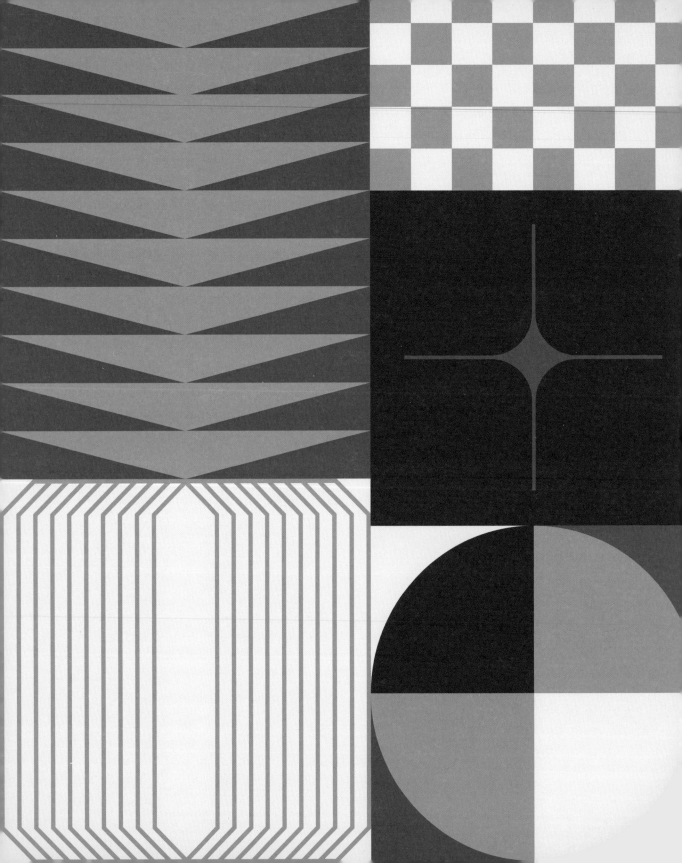

CLASSICS

RECIPES

STORIES

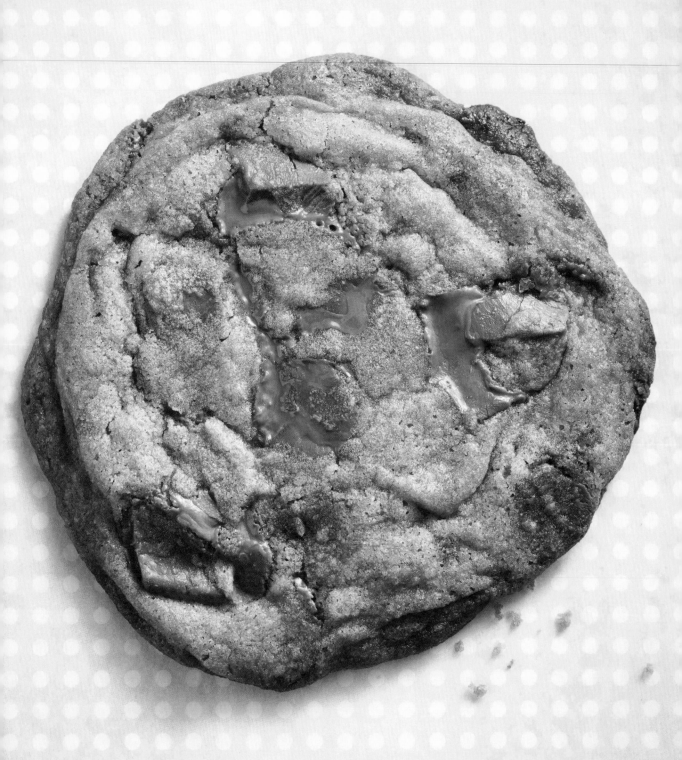

Not Just Chocolate Chip Cookies

Easier than cookies and milk.

Chocolate Chip Cookies is a balanced strain with calming effects. Just like Mom used to make, right?

Makes 21 cookies with 6 Tbsp cannabutter (about 5 mg THC per cookie).

6 Tbsp (85 g) cannabutter

½ cup + 2 Tbsp (142 g) unsalted butter, room temperature

¾ cup (150 g) brown sugar

¼ cup (50 g) granulated sugar

1 egg + 1 yolk

1 tsp vanilla extract

2 cups (284 g) all-purpose flour

1 tsp baking powder

1 tsp baking soda

Dash of salt

2 cups (340 g) high-quality chocolate chips

Preheat oven to 375°F.

Melt the cannabutter in a double boiler or in a heat-proof bowl over a pot of simmering water. Line baking sheet(s) with parchment paper.

With your favourite mixer, combine cannabutter, butter, and sugars. Add the egg, yolk, and vanilla.

In a new bowl, combine the flour, baking powder, baking soda, and salt. Add dry ingredients to the butter and sugar mixture in a few additions.

Add the chocolate chips (I like milk chocolate, but you do you).

Use a 1-Tbsp cookie scoop to drop oversized dough globs onto the prepared baking sheet(s), keeping cookies a few inches apart.

Bake in the oven for about 8 minutes. Let the cookies cool on the baking sheet(s) before moving them to a rack.

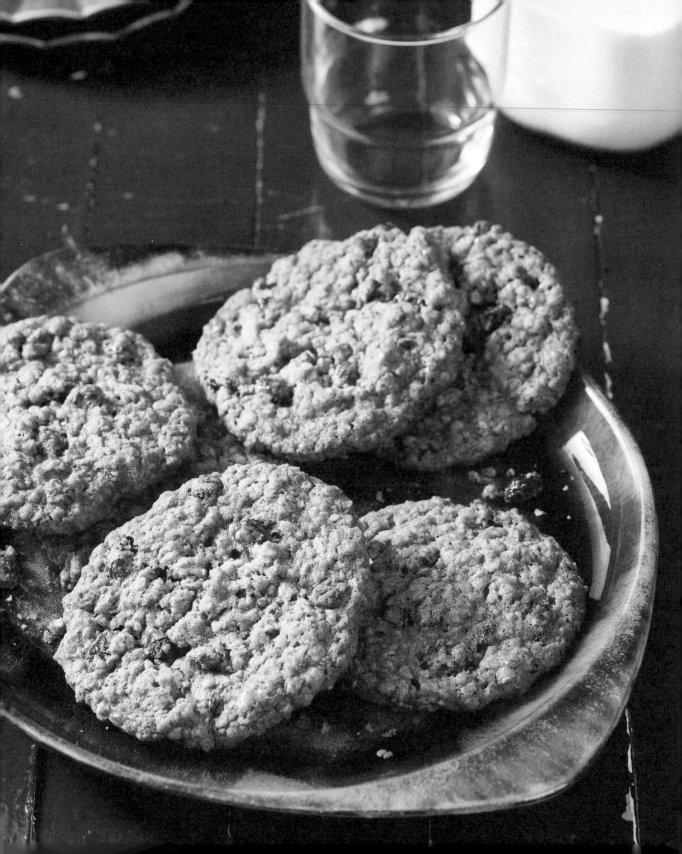

Just Right Oatmeal Raisin Cookies

As easy as just-right porridge.

SUGGESTED MOOD/STRAIN

Let's try *Grape Gas*, a balanced hybrid that smells of grapes and the earth.

Makes 27 cookies with ½ cup cannabutter (about 5 mg THC per cookie).

½ cup (113 g) cannabutter
½ cup (113 g) unsalted butter, room temperature
1 cup (200 g) brown sugar
½ cup (100 g) granulated sugar
2 eggs
1 tsp vanilla extract
1 Tbsp molasses*
1½ cups (213 g) all-purpose flour
1 tsp baking soda
1 tsp baking powder
2½ cups (200 g) quick oats
1 tsp cinnamon
Dash of salt
1½ cups (218 g) black raisins, soaked in water 10 minutes, then drained

Preheat oven to 350°F.

Melt the cannabutter in a double boiler or in a heat-proof bowl over a pot of simmering water, then cool to room temperature. Line baking sheet(s) with parchment paper.

With your favourite mixer, combine butters with sugars. Add eggs, one at a time, mixing after each addition. Add vanilla and molasses.

In a separate bowl, stir together flour, baking soda, baking powder, and oats. Add cinnamon and salt.

Add the dry ingredients to the mixing bowl. Add in the raisins. Combine.

Use a 1-Tbsp cookie scoop to lump cookie dough onto the prepared baking sheet(s). Put about six cookies on each regular-sized cookie sheet at a time.

Bake about 14 minutes, until cookies brown very slightly around the edges and are firm in the middle.

Allow cookies to cool a minute or two on the baking sheets. (Give them a bang on the counter to flatten them.) Remove to a rack to cool completely.

*Molasses: All types will work—I like strong flavour, so I went for cooking molasses. Fancy molasses is lighter. Blackstrap is the strongest and tastes bitter.

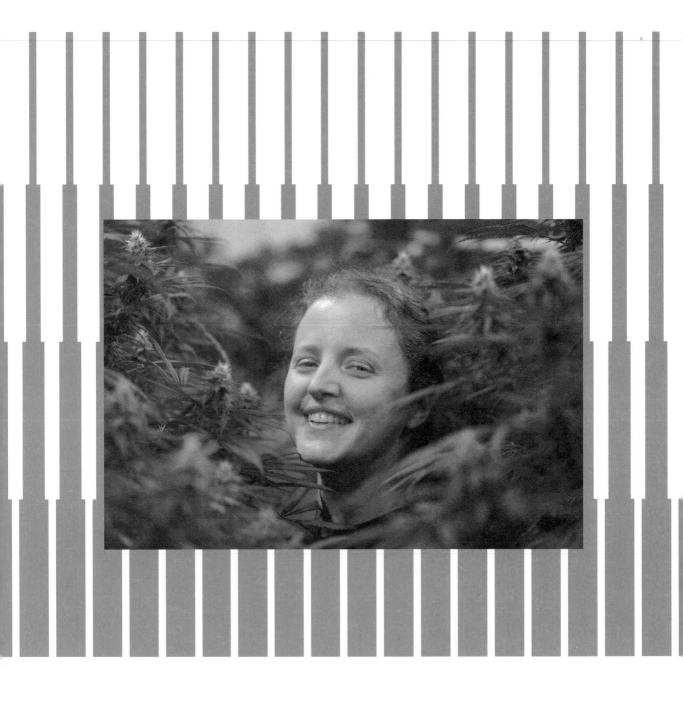

Sarah Campbell

Sarah Campbell is an herbal gardener and medicine maker based in Duncan, on Vancouver Island, in British Columbia. She works at Great Gardener Farms and is a founding director of the Craft Cannabis Association of BC. Sarah also spent years volunteering for the Vancouver Island Compassion Society (VICS), which was forced to close in 2019, despite having 3,000 members. I spoke with Sarah on her mobile while she was in the middle of a field, planting cannabis.

My history with cannabis is pretty colourful. My parents liked to smoke weed, so I became familiar with the plant at an early age. I've always been loud and proud about my cannabis use, but my first growing experience was in university. I had a few plants under an HP light under the stairs, and I had no idea what I was doing. The bud was barely smokeable, but I fell in love with those plants and really enjoyed the process. I was living in Ontario at that time, but I knew that BC was really the mecca for the cannabis movement. I told my parents that we were going to legalize cannabis one day, and they laughed, and said, "Oh yeah, we said that too, Sarah." I was serious.

I travelled to BC to visit friends in 1998 and never went home. Within a few months of being on Vancouver Island, I met Philippe Lucas, director of the Vancouver Island Compassion Society, a compassion club in Victoria. This was in the very early days of the medical cannabis movement; I believe the VICS started in 1998 and was one of just three compassion clubs in Canada. The work Philippe was doing at the VICS was incredibly inspiring, and I wanted to be a part of it—just the energy he had, and the drive to find a way for patients to have access, critically and chronically ill patients. Members were expected to die, or they had really, really severe conditions. Cannabis was often a last resort. It was about community, education, and supporting one another.

Then the VICS got robbed. And Philippe called the police. Philippe had taught kindergarten before he began this journey with cannabis—he had that schoolteacher firm will. He was a believer that he was doing nothing wrong, and he was really adamant about that. But lo and behold, after he reported the theft, I think it was the next day that the police showed up and raided the VICS, and a very lengthy court case began.

But this was the whole evolution that was necessary. Like that court case—it was one of the early high profile cannabis cases in Canada. Many witnesses travelled to testify, including senators. And the patients, too, took the stand to testify. Sick people went through that stressful experience, just to explain that this medicine was helping them with their quality of life. And in the end, the judge—Higginbotham was his name—granted Philippe an absolute discharge and praised the work being done at the VICS. It was really a beautiful thing. People from all walks of life, bound together, for this significant purpose.

And then there was the next court case. My friend at the time—life partner now, almost twenty years later—was a grower for the VICS, and he got busted for growing a thousand plants. At that time, the medical laws were that you could only grow for two other people, and he was technically growing for, like, 300 VICS members . . . I forget the numbers exactly . . . but many people. That court case took years and piles of money. These court cases were very expensive, but it was the community that came forward to ensure that they would be heard, and that they could proceed. In the end, the judge found my partner guilty, but she read out a two-hour-long decision. She said that if there was anybody who should be growing cannabis under the legal system in Canada it was him, and that there was a problem with the medical program. She concluded by saying, "Absolute discharge," and challenged Health Canada to go back to the drawing board. And so instead of being able to grow for two people, they made it so that you were able to grow for three people. And you know, that's sort of the game we've been playing with Health Canada for a long time. They'd do the bare minimum of what they had to do to satisfy the courts.

I mean, the patients are being left on the sidelines right now. The VCBC—the Victoria Cannabis Buyer's Club—is one of the last existing compassion clubs in the country. They've been raided multiple times, but they keep opening back up. They're just adamant that this model needs to exist. The VICS members voted to try and become licensed, but in the end they just couldn't do it and their doors were closed. It's a really difficult process, and you just feel like you're up against the world; it's a David and Goliath kind of thing. It's expensive, time consuming, and political. And on top of it being extremely difficult, there's

a psychological discomfort with what's happening in general. For the patients, it's like, "Where is my community? Where is anybody who cares?" The government is trying to say they're providing the patients with everything they need, but they're not *really*.

I think the future, ideally, is one where there are therapeutic centres, similar to the old compassion club model, where you have knowledgeable bud-tenders and health practitioners working together. There's a way to incorporate traditional health care with cannabis, but it's only brave doctors who are doing that at this stage. Big changes need to happen at the board level. The Canadian Medical Association— it's obviously an old guard. It's going to take a while. When you go to a recreational shop, you're basically in a bank lineup. You get moved through to the front of the line, they tell you what you need to buy, and you're out the door. Sometimes they'll chat, but it's not for the same purpose. Budtenders aren't actually allowed to talk about the benefits of the cannabis plant. We're so restricted. Even in the recreational stores, they're not allowed to talk about any kind of effects or benefits or whatever.

I think the government is reviewing the medical program now, but I don't know that they're looking at it in the best way. They're still treating it like a pharmaceutical money-making drug rather than a medicinal plant with very few negative side effects. They don't like the designated grower program. Where is their cut? Like, before legalization happened, folks in the grey market were doing everything they could to ensure clean, safe products, including testing, self-regulating, basically, and when there was extra, donations were made to ensure that people who couldn't afford the medicine could still have access. And that's still happening to some degree with substitution projects around Vancouver and in Victoria; grey market cannabis is helping people get off opiates. What a positive thing! And yet, it's like there's no support. They're still having to fight the police. The *sheer determination* of people is awe-inspiring sometimes. But yeah, it will be interesting to see what happens in the next three to five years.

But it's also been a beautiful thing, I think, for a lot of people in the country to have legalization. Around 2009, I was apprenticing with a [*non-cannabis*] herbalist. She was teaching me how to make oils and things, and that was just such a fun time, experimenting. I've met a few "wise women," I would call them. Organic gardeners, herbalists, medicine "makers." They knew my history with cannabis, of course, but they weren't comfortable, necessarily, with the idea of anything illegal. Cannabis as an herb was sort of "oh boy." So it's been interesting just seeing so many minds open to this plant that has been stuck in the underground for so long. A natural plant. And now, the makers *do* use cannabis in their oils and whatnot. I think we're going to be joining forces with the natural herbal world, in fighting for our ability to use natural medicine, and have that be okay, you know?

My focus now is to support the small-scale independent growers. In 2016, when we heard that Canada was going to legalize cannabis, a few folks in the industry—growers, retailers, consumers, policy workers—we all got together and said, "We need to make sure there's a voice for small-scale producers throughout this process." So we started the Craft Cannabis Association of BC, and we ran *the* first craft cannabis campaign in Canada. We compared the idea of craft cannabis to craft beer. We promoted the idea that small-scale independents were the source of quality cannabis, and that regionality and knowing your farmer are just as appealing as with other local products.

We worked with the government at every opportunity to provide feedback. We have several papers on our website. We gave our perspective. And now, we're very focused on British Columbia. We've established, after three or four years, good relationships with regulators in the province, and we're working to establish an official category for craft cannabis. Like craft beer, we've defined craft cannabis as small scale, independent, and artisanal. There's this little war happening between us and Ontario, for example. Ontario wants to take this big approach allowing large companies to acquire a craft label. But from our perspective, it's very much about small independent businesses. I think the small guys are the ones that actually need the support. This is where consumers are going—ethical consumption, regionality, locality. Everyone wants to call themselves "craft," and so, yeah, we're sticking to our guns at this point.

I really believe, though, that within a few years, we're going to be on the right track. A good track. It's very difficult right now for the small producers. There are so many fingers in the pie that it's really hard to make a living. But I'm optimistic that the regulations will be relaxed at some point, to some degree. We need to create an industry that people want to become a part of. And then I hope that the patients have a program that all of us in Canada can be proud of. We were the first country to do this on a very large scale, and we've always said, let's be the example.

Craft cannabis exists and supports communities in every country of the world. It's grassroots. And if people lose the ability to contribute to the health and well-being of their local communities because legalization has come along, everybody's going to be in trouble. Hopefully, we'll find a way for craft growers' roles within their communities to be acknowledged and appreciated. The transition to legalization in Canada is proving to be a difficult one, but I have faith. Grassroots movements are the real deal.

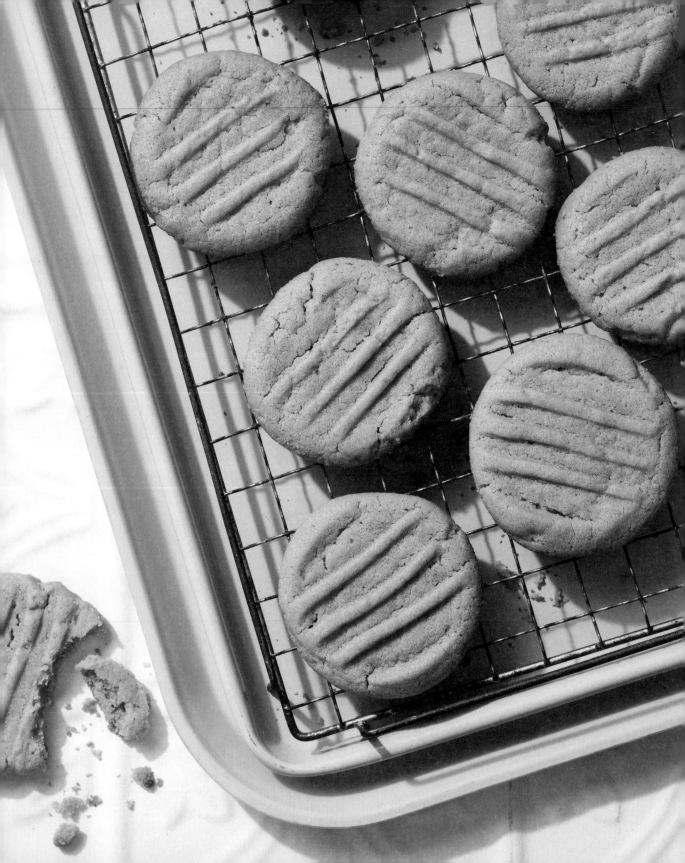

Gram's Peanut Butter Cookies

This recipe is easier than gulping after biting off more PB than you can chew. This was my grandmother's peanut butter cookie recipe, and she definitely would not have been a pot smoker. I've infused it and will share it with you guys, but doing so may mean I'll get yelled at forever in the afterlife. You're worth it.

SUGGESTED MOOD/STRAIN

Let's go with *Peanut Butter Breath*, a sedating hybrid with a nutty smell.

Makes 24 cookies with ½ cup cannabutter (about 6 mg THC per cookie).

½ cup (113 g) cannabutter
Cooking spray
1 cup (200 g) granulated sugar
1 cup (200 g) brown sugar
½ cup (113 g) lard (or shortening),
   room temperature
1 egg
1 tsp vanilla extract
1 cup (280 g) peanut butter
2 cups (284 g) all-purpose flour
1 tsp baking soda
Dash of salt

Preheat oven to 350°F.

Melt the cannabutter in a double boiler or in a heat-proof bowl over a pot of simmering water, and prepare baking sheet(s) with cooking spray.

With your favourite mixer, combine cannabutter, sugars, and lard. Add the egg, vanilla, and peanut butter.

In another bowl, stir together flour, baking soda, and salt. Add the dry ingredients to the mixing bowl.

Using a 1-Tbsp cookie scoop, measure scoops of dough and roll them into balls. Set the balls onto baking sheet(s) and squash them gently with a large serving fork; they won't spread too much beyond this size.

Bake cookies until crisp, about 15 minutes. Now, these cookies are delicate, so let them rest on the cookie sheet(s) about 5 minutes, then move them to a rack with a flat spatula. (They'll crumble if you move them too quickly; don't ask how I know.) Let cookies cool completely before serving.

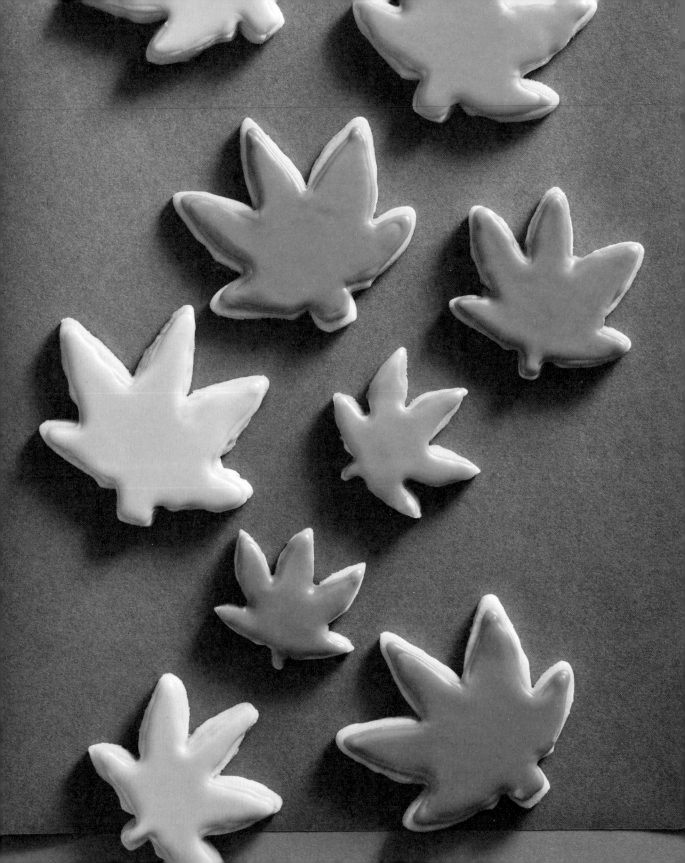

Cut Outs

This recipe is easier than explaining that it's cannabis leaves and not mistletoe that you've contributed to the Christmas cookie exchange (and yet everyone is shocked that they're somehow getting kissed more).

SUGGESTED MOOD/STRAIN

Let's go with *Zookies*, a hybrid strain that helps bypass the couch.

Makes about 26 (3 × 4–inch) leaves with ½ cup cannabutter (over 5 mg THC per cookie).

Cookies

½ cup (113 g) cannabutter
½ cup (113 g) unsalted butter,
   room temperature
1 cup (200 g) granulated sugar
1 egg
1 tsp vanilla extract
3 cups (426 g) all-purpose flour
1 tsp baking powder
1 tsp cornstarch
A few dashes of salt

Icing

7 Tbsp pasteurized egg whites +
   more if needed*
5½ cups icing (powdered) sugar (622 g)
   + more as needed, sifted through
   a fine mesh sieve
3 gel colours of your choice

To make the cookies: Melt the cannabutter in a double boiler or in a heat-proof bowl over a pot of simmering water, then cool to room temperature.

With your favourite mixer, combine the butters and sugar. Add the egg and vanilla.

In a separate bowl, mix the dry ingredients with a wooden spoon (flour, baking powder, cornstarch, and salt). Add the dry ingredients to the mixing bowl, letting the dough come together. Divide the dough into two lumps, flatten, and cover in plastic wrap. Refrigerate for at least an hour.

Preheat the oven to 350°F and line baking sheet(s) with parchment paper or silicone mat(s). Remove a dough lump from the fridge, and toss plastic wrap. Sandwich the dough between two pieces of parchment, and roll it out to about ¼-inch thick. This will take a bit of muscle, but you can handle it. With cookie cutter(s), cut out as many leaves (or other shapes) as you can and set them on the baking sheets, about an inch apart.

Mash the dough bits together, roll the lump out, and cut more shapes. Repeat until there's just a wee bit of dough left. Repeat with the other refrigerated disk (but only with as many cookies as your baking sheets and oven can handle at once). Keep the rest of the dough refrigerated until ready for use.

Bake for about 8–10 minutes until the cookies are very gently brown around the edges. Allow the cookies to cool completely on a rack before decorating.

To decorate: Pasteurize your egg whites so that no one confuses salmonella poisoning for cannabis effects.

Prepare a big batch of icing by combining the icing sugar

and egg whites in a medium size bowl, and then cover it with a damp towel. (Icing is the right consistency if you cut a knife through it and it takes about eight seconds to come back together. Add more egg whites or icing sugar if needed.) Divide the icing between three small bowls, and add a few drops of gel colouring to each as you like.

Cut about an inch off the end of a piping bag and set it up with a small round tip (#1.5). Set the icing bag into a tall glass and fold the wide part of the bag inside-out over the glass. Use a silicone spatula to fill the bag with one of the icings, and then close the top of the bag, forcing the icing down into the tip. Give the consistency a little try (not on a cookie) to make sure it pipes well. Or, if you prefer to use a squeeze bottle, use a funnel to fill one.

Pipe the edge of a cookie by touching the decorating tip to the cookie surface to start, and then holding the piping bag mid-air above the cookie, letting the icing fall, all the way around the cookie's border. Dollop more of the icing onto the cookie with a spoon and tease it out just over the border line using a new paint brush or toothpick, to flood the surface of the cookie. Finish ⅓ of the cookies with that colour. Repeat with the other icing colours, washing the decorating tip in between (unless you're a lucky b$stard who owns more). Let the cookies set for at least an hour, or preferably overnight.

*Buying egg whites in a carton lets you skip the pasteurization step with the icing. If using regular eggs, heat water to 140–142°F, remove the water from the heat, and put room-temperature eggs in the bath for 3½ minutes before separating them (they'll stay raw at that temp). If your eggs weren't room temperature, place them in a bowl of warm water for a few minutes prior to their legit bath.

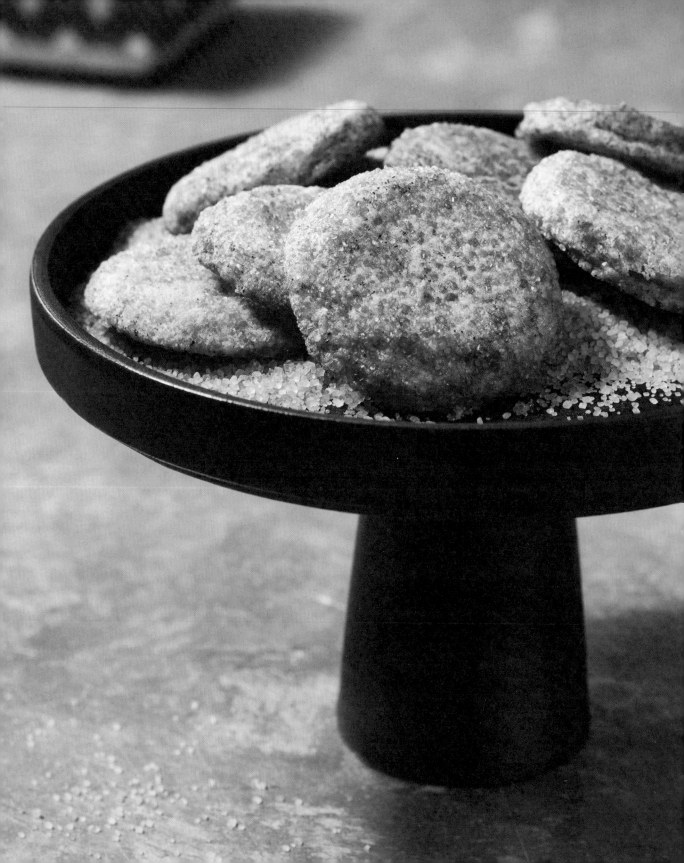

Gluten-Free Snickerdoodles

Easier than inventing the word "snickerdoodle."

Let's go with *Cinnamon Twist*, an indica-dominant strain that smells like
. . . guess what?

Makes 25 cookies with ½ cup cannabutter (almost 6 mg THC per cookie).

½ cup (113 g) cannabutter

½ cup (113 g) unsalted regular butter, room temperature

1¼ cups (250 g) granulated sugar

2 eggs

2 tsp vanilla extract

2½ cups (500 g) gluten-free flour*

2 tsp cream of tartar (white powder, stoner, not liquid cream)

1 tsp baking soda

2 tsp cinnamon, divided

Dash of salt

¼ cup (50 g) turbinado (coarse) sugar

Preheat oven to 375°F.

Melt the cannabutter in a double boiler or in a heat-proof bowl over a pot of simmering water. Line your baking sheet(s) with parchment paper.

With your favourite mixer, combine cannabutter, butter, and sugar. Add the eggs, one by one, and then the vanilla.

In a separate bowl, stir the dry ingredients (gluten-free flour, cream of tartar, baking soda, 1 tsp cinnamon, and salt). Add the dry ingredients to the mixing bowl.

In a small bowl, combine the reserved 1 tsp cinnamon with the turbinado sugar. Set aside.

This is quite a gooey batter, but you're going to get all up in there. Don't worry, it's somehow cathartic. Work out some little balls (about 1 Tbsp; add a bit more flour if it's too hard to work with) and then roll them well in the turbinado/cinnamon mixture. These cookies will spread a fair bit, so make sure they're spaced well apart on the baking sheet(s).

Bake in preheated oven about 8 minutes. The cookies are finished when they start to look flat around the edge and are a little crackly, but are slightly domed in the centre. (They'll flatten as they cool.)

Give the baking sheets a smack on the counter, and let the cookies rest to cool completely before moving (or the little bastards will fall apart).

*Gluten-free flour: Double-check to make sure this includes xanthan gum. If it doesn't, add ½ tsp.

Leonardo Oliveira

Leo Oliveira is a writer who immigrated to Toronto from São Paulo, Brazil, when he was twenty-five, in 2009. I'm grateful to be able to call him a friend.

I've always been the kid who really wanted to experience the world for myself. I came out when I was sixteen, and I was very certain about my sexual orientation and queer spirit. It wasn't like, "Oh, I want to talk to you about this" with my parents; I just came out. And not only were they not very accepting, but a lot of other bad things were also happening at that same time, especially at school. So it didn't come as a surprise to me when I first experimented with cannabis in college. What surprised me was how the experience would help me become a more positive and resilient person.

I have always dealt with bad/traumatic experiences by myself. Bullying at school, sexual abuse, and physical assault are the worst examples. And dealing with feelings that came from those experiences by myself was quite harmful. It all drove me to the mental state I was in at the age of twenty-one, which culminated in me surviving suicide. But we're here to talk about cannabis, right?

So I was twenty-one when I had my first experience with pot. I was at college [*in Brazil*], and at the time, I smoked a joint. The quality of any kind of product that we were getting in Latin America was not the best. It's a block, basically. A brick. You don't even know what's in it, and the only way you can get it is illegally. Even though there was kind of a movement toward legalization at one point, around 2009, a lot of conservatives went into the government, especially from the church, specifically, the evangelical church, and they stopped everything. With this president [*Jair Bolsonaro*], all the conversations that had been happening, they were just burned, to be honest, and cannabis went back into a drug that is used to reinforce racial discrimination, police brutality, and the prison system.

So, that time in 2009, when I was twenty-one, was a very troubling period for me. And cannabis helped put me in a state of relaxation and contemplation a little bit more. So the use, even though I didn't know much about it, started to be more medicinal for me, at the time, controlling a lot of the negative thoughts that were going on, especially related to burnout from work and university. Right now I can look in hindsight at when I started and see that I was in a horrible, horrible pattern. But when I started smoking pot, my emotional reactions became more controllable. I was able to mediate myself much better, into what was a more positive way of thinking, and away from a negative way of thinking.

Since I've immigrated to Canada, I've been very, very lucky for having many opportunities that I know other people wouldn't have. Like joining a therapy program promoted by the University of Toronto that was free of charge and having the incredible love and support of my soon-to-be husband when times were the hardest. I've reconciled with my past

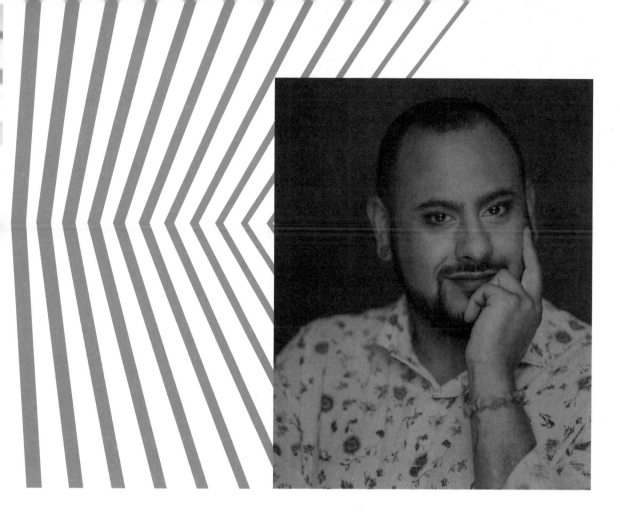

and my family and simply learned a lot from the immigration experience. I am very grateful for how I am able to have more of a mature point of view about everything, especially when it comes to cannabis use.

So, despite a lot of things that happened, in terms of trauma and events and family relationships, I believe that cannabis, as a whole, allows me to interact with my reality in a more grounded and positive way. Overall, the beginning of the road for me was very turbulent, but it's nice to be able to see myself in a calmer, more positive, and healthier state, and know that cannabis was not something that deterred me from my objectives, like, for example, alcohol was very close to doing.

Nowadays, I also enjoy spending relaxing times at a park or on a beach after I have one of the cookies I bake myself. I learned to make butter, use better doses, and become more mindful of how I am treating and loving myself.

Bringing together the information as to how the mind works and knowing that cannabis helped me was very much necessary for me to not demonize myself for using a substance that in many countries is still illegal. It's been a long time. There's definitely been a lot of work done, which is great. And although the work is still far from over when it comes to my journey, nowadays I can say I am truly happy.

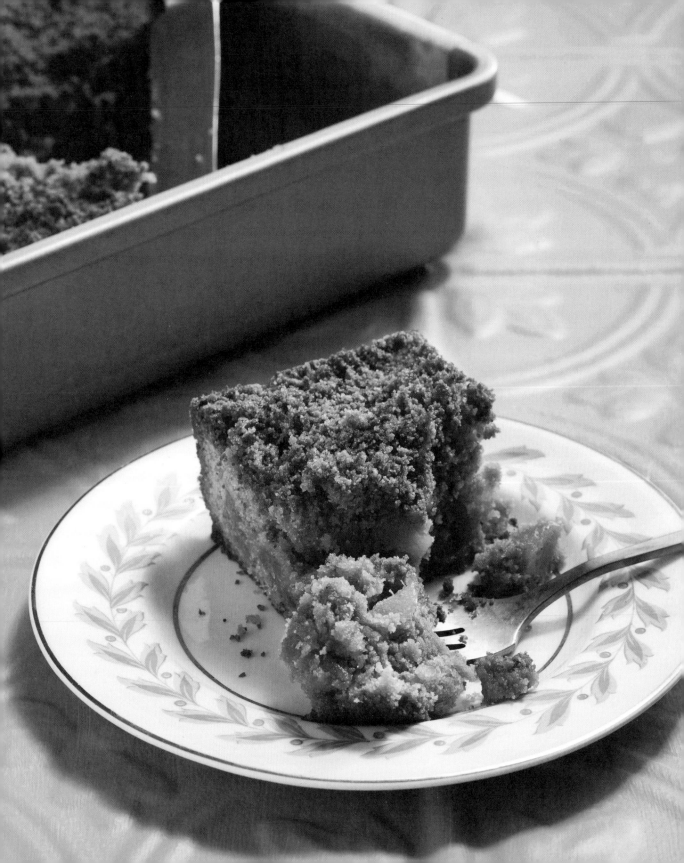

Gingersnap Blondies

This recipe is easier than keeping up with the sunscreen if you're a ginger.

SUGGESTED MOOD/STRAIN
Ginger Punch is a hybrid that's said to smell like strawberry candy.

Makes 16 squares with 6 Tbsp cannabutter (almost 7 mg THC per piece).

¼ cup + 2 Tbsp cannabutter (85 g)

½ cup + 2 Tbsp unsalted butter (142 g) at room temperature, divided

1¾ cups + 3 Tbsp (388 g) brown sugar, divided

2 eggs

2 cups (284 g) all-purpose flour

1 tsp baking powder

Dash of salt

1 Tbsp vanilla extract

1 cup (150 g) finely diced candied ginger (sorry, this process is annoying but it's worth it)

3 store-bought gingersnap cookies (about 2 inches in diameter), pulsed into crumbs in a food processor (aiming for 60 g of crumbs, in case your snaps should differ from 2 inches)

Preheat oven to 350°F.

Melt the cannabutter in a double boiler or in a heat-proof bowl over a pot of simmering water. Prepare an 8 × 8–inch* square pan with parchment across the bottom and up two of the sides (to be used as handles).

With your favourite mixer, combine the cannabutter, ½ cup butter, and 1¾ cups brown sugar. Add the eggs, one at a time.

In a separate bowl, stir together the flour, baking powder, and salt. Add to the mixing bowl. Add the vanilla.

Add in the candied ginger. Pour the batter into the pan.

With a food processor, whiz together the gingersnaps, remaining 2 Tbsp butter, and reserved 3 Tbsp brown sugar. Sprinkle over the top of the batter.

Bake your blondies, checking after 40 minutes. If you tap the centre and it jiggles like my post-COVID stomach, return to the oven, checking every 5 minutes until the middle firms up.

Allow the blondies to cool to warm, then chill completely in the fridge. Lift the block onto a flat surface with the parchment handles and slice it into quarters, and then quarters again (16 pieces).

*If you have a 9 × 9–inch pan, increase ingredients by 25 percent.

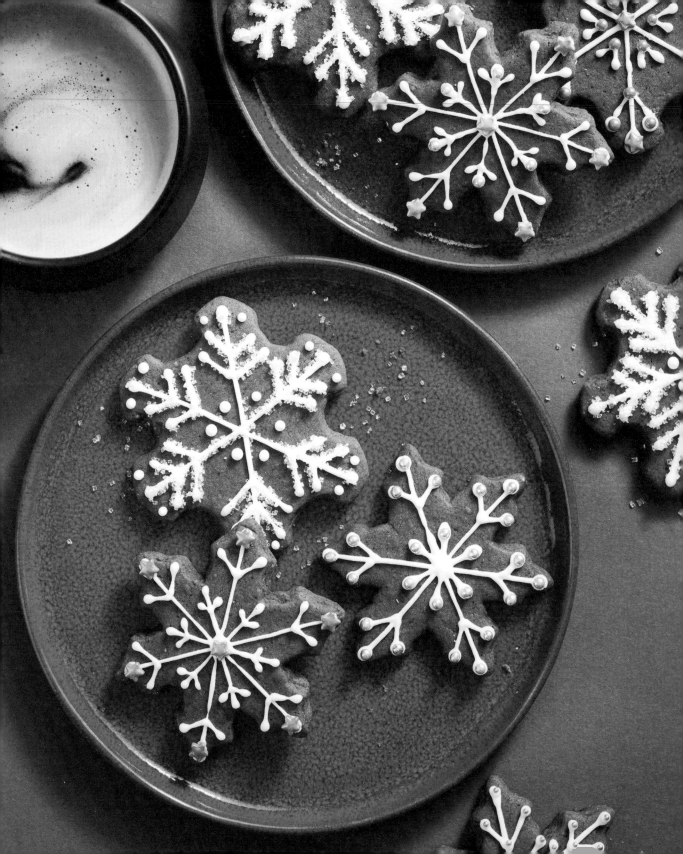

Gingerbread Snowflakes

This recipe is easier than chasing down that damn gingerbread man.
(Let's be real—a stoner couldn't even be bothered.)

SUGGESTED MOOD/STRAIN

Snow Bud is a sativa-dominant hybrid named for its thick, snowy-looking resin.

Makes 30 snowflakes with ½ cup cannabutter + 2 Tbsp (about 6 mg THC per cookie).

Cookies

½ cup + 2 Tbsp (142 g) cannabutter

2 Tbsp unsalted butter (29 g), melted

¾ cup (150 g) brown sugar

⅓ cup molasses*

1 egg

2 cups (284 g) all-purpose flour

¾ cup (117 g) whole wheat flour

2 Tbsp ginger

2 tsp cinnamon

½ tsp allspice

¼ tsp nutmeg

1 tsp baking soda

Dash of salt

Icing

2½ cups (283 g) icing (powdered) sugar, sifted

½ tsp vanilla extract

2 Tbsp milk

Pretty little ball decorations and/or sprinkles

To make the cookies: Melt the cannabutter in a double boiler or in a heat-proof bowl over a pot of simmering water.

With your favourite mixer, combine the butters and brown sugar. Add the molasses and the egg.

In a separate bowl, mix the flours, spices, baking soda, and salt. Add these to the mixing bowl in a few additions. Split the dough in half, flatten each blob into a disk, cover in plastic wrap, and refrigerate for at least an hour.

Preheat oven to 350°F. Line baking sheet(s) with parchment paper. Roll out one of the dough disks with your rolling pin between two sheets (more) parchment, to about ¼-inch thick. Cut your snowflakes with a 3-inch snowflake cookie cutter or two and place them on the baking sheet(s). Mash the remaining dough bits together and roll the dough again, cutting more flakes. Repeat until there's no dough left, and do the same with the other doughy disk.

Bake your flakes for about 8 minutes, until they've lost their shine and are firm to the touch. After a minute or so out of the oven, remove them to a rack to cool completely.

To decorate: Whisk the icing sugar, vanilla, and milk together. You know the icing is about right if it has a toothpaste consistency. Go ahead and cover the bowl with a wet tea towel or plastic wrap to keep it from going crispy as you use it.

Cut about an inch off the end of a piping bag and set it up with a small round tip (#1.5). Set the icing bag into a tall glass and fold the wide part of the bag inside-out over the glass. Use a silicone spatula to fill the bag with the outline icing, and then close the top of the bag, forcing the icing down into the tip. Give the consistency a little try (not on a cookie) to make sure it pipes a pretty line.

Decorate the surface of each cookie with pretty lines, curlicues, and dots. If you mess something up, slide a piece of paper under the icing line and lift the mistake away, never to be seen or heard from again. Decorate with little pretty balls (tee-hee), if you like. Continue, until you get a batch of gorgeous buzzy snowflakes. Catch one on your tongue.

*Molasses: All types will work—I like strong flavour, so I went for cooking molasses. Fancy molasses is lighter. Blackstrap is the strongest and tastes bitter.

Dave Belisle

Dave Belisle is the owner of the Medicine Box, a medicinally minded cannabis dispensary in Kanesatake, a Mohawk settlement in southwestern Quebec. Dave has a bachelor's degree in Aboriginal social work and a degree in community diabetes work. He's worked in Kanesatake for fifteen years as a community worker, youth worker, and with the National Native Alcohol & Drug Addiction Program.

Before reading Dave's story, I encourage you to check out Sarah Campbell's interview (see page 39). Dave and Sarah are cannabis practitioners who have never met and who live across the country from each other. But Sarah identifies a gap in the current medicinal cannabis care model where patients are left with limited options beyond using recreational dispensaries. Dave has intuitively stepped up to try to fulfill this need in his community. The Medicine Box works to heal its clients using cannabis holistically; its staff takes the time to understand the physical, psychological, and cultural needs of the entire person.

My philosophy is, yeah, cannabis could be a gateway drug, but it's a gateway to healing, to curing, and everything else.

[Hey, it's an "Ann's two cents" moment! The gateway theory as it relates to drug use has been disproven by scientists, not just Dave. Many who use "harder" drugs have tried cannabis, but most who have used weed do not move on to harder drugs. Drug experimentation and addiction are complicated, where factors may include risk tolerance, genetics, mental health, trauma, and other contributors.]

I've always dabbled in marijuana. I've grown it every year, and I've always understood the medicinal values. I really got stuck with all the stigmas from the older generation who might now be in their late fifties to seventies, though, about being a smoker; that I wasn't going to make it anywhere, and that cannabis was going to make me brain dead. Those thoughts played at the back of my mind, but I still got a university degree. I went to school for "Aboriginal approach to social work." My degree was in social work, sure, but it also included incorporation of ceremonies and how to counsel using our traditional medicines to help people through their ailments.

Also, for me personally, cannabis has helped me reach sobriety. I've been two years sober, not a drop of alcohol, and that's thanks to cannabis. I use edibles at night to sleep. I smoke on a daily basis. I'm healthy, I have no diabetes, and I have no chronic ailments. I wouldn't say that's all from cannabis, but it has a lot to do with it.

And that's not the only success story about marijuana. I have many friends and clients who are free of opioid addictions because of cannabis. It's helping a lot of people. It should have gone legal a long time ago.

Let's fast-forward a bit to starting the business.

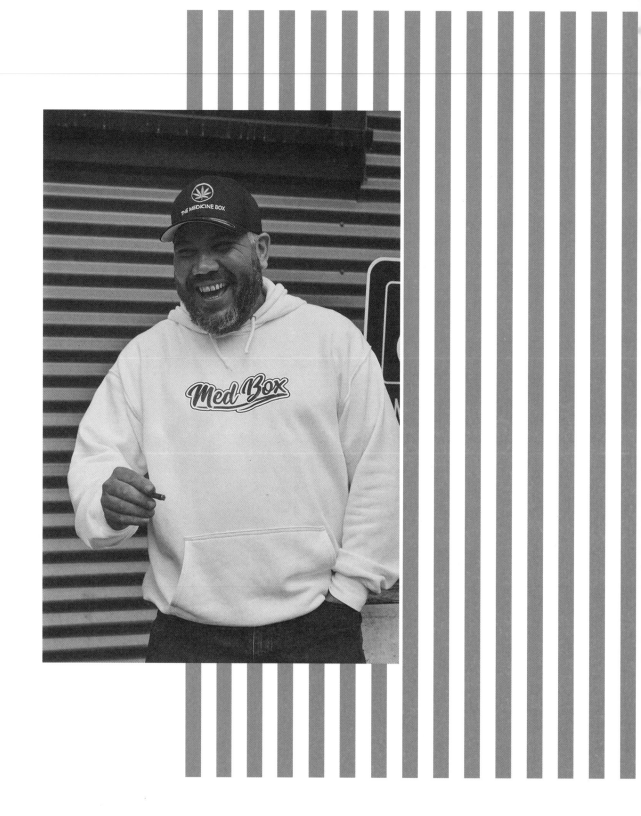

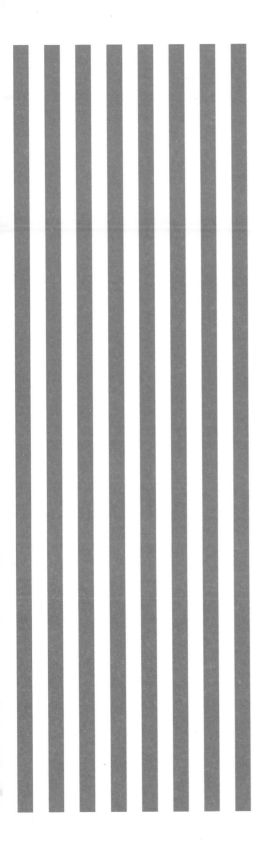

When cannabis became legal, I knew that opening the store was something I wanted to do, just because of my social work background and counselling. I knew that there was a way that I could link cannabis and the two together to work out the stigma and improve the education about it. So I started working on cannabis education. There wasn't much at the time; there were very few studies out there. Every study that was done looked for the negative effects, never the positive. So it was a little hard.

When we got into the business, there were already two shops in the community. We knew we wanted to take a different approach, to make it more medicinal, more accessible, and have more products, where it's not just the cannabis in the flower form, but everything for every purpose. Like with CBD, we have CBD drops, coffee, and tinctures. We have CBD gummies, capsules, and even suppositories. We have full-spectrum CBD, which is THC, THCA, CBD, and CBN—everything from the plant.

Our name, The Medicine Box, was something of the older people. A medicine chest would have been used by the people in the past.

We opened our shop out of a shipping container on December 7, 2019. We didn't know how it was going to be. The laws were fresh; it was fresh in Canada, being legal for just over a year. The dispensaries here, like I said, there were only two running. And it was in a grey zone, and ad hoc, pretty much, because the Band Council didn't know what to do. The government was like, "Well, it's up to Council."

We had a lot of hurdles to overcome, but we did it.

[From Ann: I've read about some dispensaries on reserve—not Kanesatake—but that they've been raided by the RCMP. Is that a conflict in jurisdiction?]

Yes, but the thing is, too, a lot of times when raids happen in the communities, there's a little note that goes out to the Council saying something like, "This is what's happening in the Community. We have to come in and regulate this." Our Council was approached a few times by the RCMP and the SQ [*the Sûreté du Québec, the Québec provincial police*] and the Council said, "No, you can't do anything. This is an internal matter and we'll work it out ourselves."

To this day, there's still not clear regulation, but we're getting there. When we opened our doors, like I said, we were in a small shipping container. Within a week, we had a lineup out the door. Within two months, we had a little fire that forced us to get into a bigger building. After that, it really just opened up. We have clients that are from eighteen to ninety-two that come in. And it's pretty surprising because some of the older ones smoked when they were younger, but now they're trying to start again, and it's helping them move around, it's making them more active, it's helping them sleep at night. So they're really rediscovering the benefits of cannabis use.

We have a wide variety of people that come in from all walks of life. And that's what we try to cater to. We have patients with Crohn's disease. We have MMA fighters coming in for their body ailments. I have tattoo artists that are coming in for our salves because it's helping them heal faster, and it's helping the pain. Yes, cannabis is recreational now, but the more cannabis products we have, the more people we can help. Because not everybody takes THC, and not everyone goes for CBD. Some smoke for pleasure, while others smoke for actual medicating reasons.

Right now, we're linked with other First Nations communities for most of our supply, but we also grow our own. We work with a large network of different First Nations communities that have already established their own products. We also have our own

in-lab testing, including full spectrometer testing, 3-phase toxicity tests, testing for mould, pesticides, herbicides—anything that could be harmful for human consumption. And we got those testing capabilities within the first year of opening because we wanted to make our name and be true to what we sell.

Maybe most importantly, we offer one-on-ones. I worked for fifteen years in the local health centre, run by Health Canada. They supported me and sent me through all kinds of education, and I'm so grateful for it, because I got to apply it in my last job. But now I can really get into it, to help a spectrum of people, to see the differences in them, and to bring the happiness back.

We have people coming in that just recently learned they have cancer. They know they're going to die. But we're helping them live their better lives. They want to go to a place where they're going to feel comfort, where they're going to feel that somebody cares and is going to take the time to help them get through it. That's what we take the time to do, and I think that my social work experiences and counselling experiences help with that. We can help them through depression, anxiety, and whatever else they might need.

I took a community diabetes prevention program, and that also helped me in the field I'm in, because now we offer vegan products, sugar-free products, and I can get to the one-on-ones with people who are going through neuropathy, which is the nerve damage in their feet and hands. I can suggest different cannabis products that will help them to get the sensation back, or some of the tingling back, or help them to relax.

Another thing is that all of our staff is educated in what could affect some of the common medications. Like high blood pressure pills, for example. High blood pressure pills are made to reduce your blood pressure, but CBD can also open up your blood vessels. So you could double react with your medication.

I think that's what the government places are lacking. If you go into a place like that, you can't really talk to a person. In the SQDC [*the Société Québécoise du Cannabis, which has a legislated monopoly on the sale of recreational cannabis in Québec*], you can't just walk in and say, "Hey, I've got this. What can you help me with?" They can't tell you anything.

Let's say somebody is a very anxious person and you sell them sativa. You just made their anxiety go 110 percent, through the roof. And then there are the terpene profiles. The terpenes have a lot to do with how you get your high, how your high is delivered, or how the effects are delivered to your body. The SQDC doesn't explain that either. Crazy little things like that.

It wasn't intentionally that we started treating more than just the cannabis needs, it just came out, as in nature. We had a family member of a patient that came into the store just last month and they'd tried everything. Their father was in the hospital, he wasn't eating, he was in pain, he was living his worst days of the cancer. His dying days. And they came to us, and the lady cried in my arms. "I don't know what to do anymore," she cried, and you could see the frustration in her eyes. She released about how her family member was in the hospital, how he wasn't sleeping, in constant pain, that the minute they touched him, it felt like his skin was on fire. We started going through and talking and talking, and then we suggested some products that might help him.

Yes, we sell recreational products, but for those people that are really looking for a new alternative to healing, we can educate them through that, too. I mean, we've been open for, it's going to be, three years. We've had some staff come and go, but lately the last almost year and a half, it's been the same staff, and they are phenomenal. They really wear their hearts on their sleeves. And I think that's what keeps our customers coming back, too. I say customers loosely—I'd rather say clients. At some point, we've made new friends.

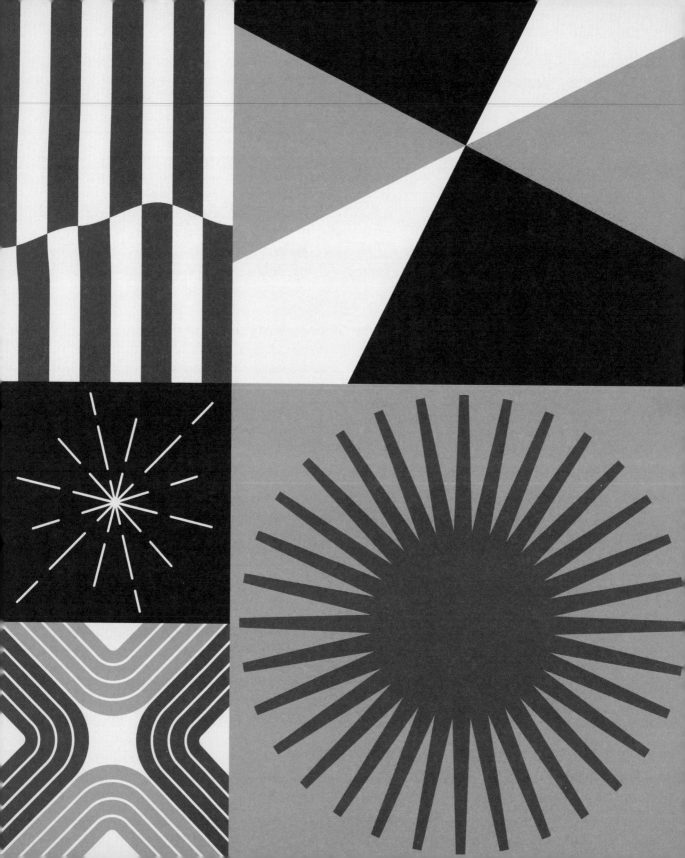

CHOCOLATE

RECIPES

STORIES

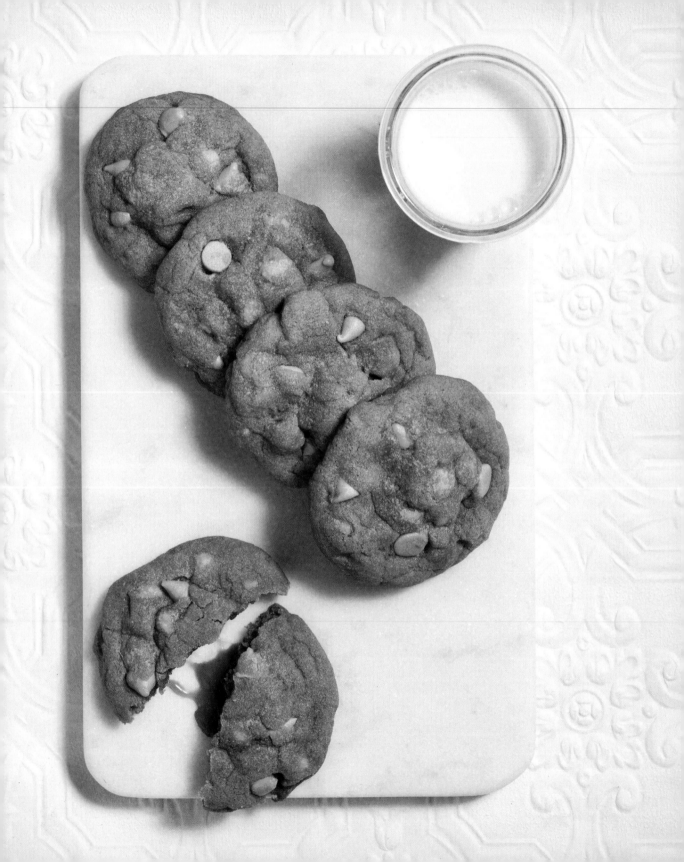

Brown Butter Rolo Cookies

This recipe is easier than rolling a Rolo to your pal. And potentially getting sued for using a brand name in a pot cookie book. Hey, when I say "Rolo" from here on in, I'm talking about generic chocolate-covered, soft caramel-like candies that may or may not roll down your driveway in their packaging. Mmmkay?

SUGGESTED MOOD/STRAIN

Let's go with *Bolo*, mostly because it rhymes with Rolo. *Bolo* is a 50/50 hybrid. The cool kids tell me that *Bolo* stands for "Be on the lookout." But the fact that I know that means it's probably not the cool kids who are saying that.

Makes about 26 cookies with ½ cup cannabutter (over 5 mg THC per cookie).

Cooking spray
½ cup (113 g) cannabutter
½ cup (113 g) unsalted butter
2½ cups (355 g) all-purpose flour
1 tsp baking soda
Dash of salt
1½ cups (330 g) packed brown sugar
1 egg + 1 yolk
1 tsp vanilla extract
1 cup (170 g) butterscotch chips
26 "Rolos"*

Preheat oven to 350°F and prepare baking sheet(s) with cooking spray. Melt cannabutter in a double boiler or in a heat-proof bowl over a pot of simmering water. In a small heavy-bottomed pot, melt the regular butter over medium-low heat, whisking occasionally, until it stops bubbling, looks foamy, and begins to brown (about 8 minutes). If you nailed it, the wee saucepan will smell extra buttery (if it goes black, go through a moment or two of self-loathing, toss it, and try again). Allow the butters to cool a little.

While your cow fats are cooling, in a new bowl, combine the flour, baking soda, and salt. Set aside.

Using your favourite mixer, combine butters and sugar. Add the egg, yolk, and vanilla, and mix until smooth.

Add the dry ingredients to the mixing bowl in two additions.

Using a wooden spoon (or a mixer at slow speed if you're lazy, like me), fold in the butterscotch chips.

Use a 1-Tbsp cookie scoop to drop dough globs onto the baking sheet(s), and tuck a Rolo inside each one, making sure each chocolate is surrounded with dough. Space the cookies at least 2 inches apart.

Bake in a preheated oven for about 7 minutes. Smack the baking sheet(s) a few times and allow the cookies to cool for a couple of minutes before transferring them to a wire rack to cool completely.

*The recipe calls for 26 "Rolos": There are 10 chocolates in a package, so buy 3 packages and eat the 4 leftover chocolates.

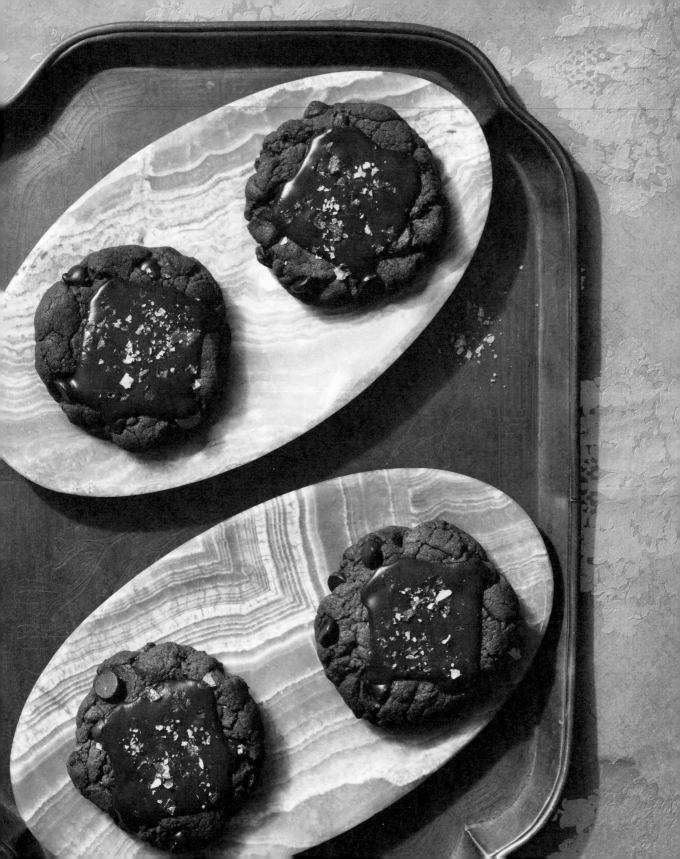

Triple Chocolate Cookies

Easier than Augustus Gloop falling into the chocolate river.

Chocolope Kush is a sativa-dominant strain that derives from the lineage of *Chocolope* and *Kosher Kush*.

Makes 21 cookies with ½ cup cannabutter (almost 7 mg THC per cookie).

½ cup (113 g) cannabutter
¼ cup (57 g) unsalted butter
½ cup (100 g) granulated sugar
½ cup (100 g) brown sugar
2 eggs
1 tsp baking soda
½ tsp baking powder
2 cups (284 g) all-purpose flour
½ cup (43 g) cocoa powder
Dash of salt
1¼ cups (213 g) dark chocolate chips
21 flat chocolate squares (sectioned from bars) of your choice*
Flaky sea salt

Preheat oven to 350°F and line baking sheet(s) with parchment paper or silicone mat(s).

Melt the butters in a double boiler or in a heat-proof bowl over a pot of simmering water. Let them cool a titch, and add to the bowl of your favourite mixer.

Add in the sugars and eggs and mix well.

In a separate bowl, mix the baking soda, baking powder, flour, cocoa, and a dash of salt.

Add the dry ingredients to the mixing bowl. Mix in the chips. Using a 1-Tbsp cookie scoop, spoon generous dollops of dough onto the baking sheet(s), and manhandle them into chubby cookies. Top each with a chocolate square.

Bake about 6 minutes, until the chocolate is glistening and the cookie has lost its shine. Remove, smacking the cookie sheet on the counter to settle the chocolate. Sprinkle with sea salt. Let the cookies cool completely and sprinkle a titch more salt.

Find some milk.

*For the flat gourmet chocolate bars broken into squares, I like the ones that rhyme with "splint." From Switzerland. No, not those ones, different ones. I'm not going to get sued, you're going to get sued. Anyway, pick a type you like the flavour profile of. I like dark chocolate with sea salt.

Audrey McEwan

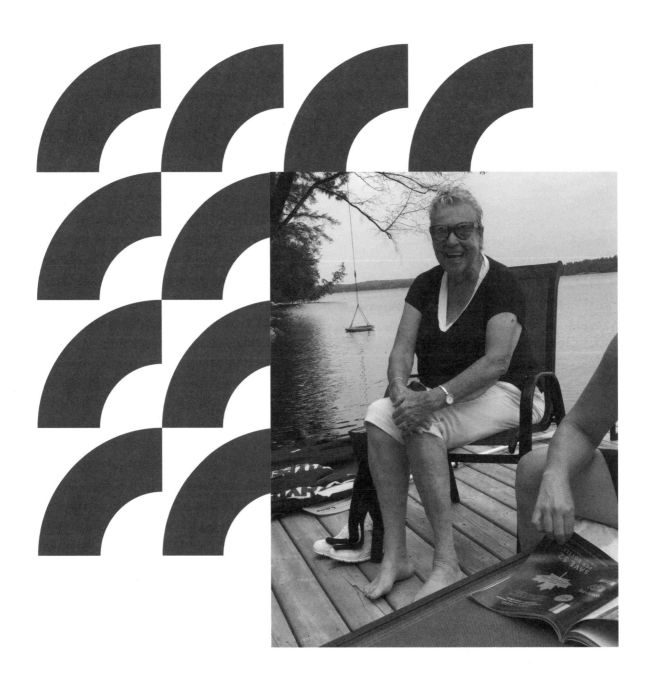

Audrey McEwen, now based in Calgary, Alberta, with eighty-one feisty years under her belt, was a nurse by trade before her retirement. While I haven't had the pleasure of meeting many of the interviewees for this book, I have been lucky enough to spend time with Aud, as she's my friend's aunt. We were lakeside when she shared her story of going to prison in Amsterdam for six months for smuggling hash from India. I asked Aud to retell the story for me here, and she graciously obliged.

Although I've always been a big reader and love how stories come across in writing, in this case, I wish you could hear Aud's actual voice. As you read, please picture her story told in her careful, thoughtful drawl, interrupted occasionally by her slow laugh. Composed, mischievous Aud calling herself a "drug mule" will just never come across properly in black and white. C'est la vie.

Well, I don't have any qualms at all about sharing my story. This happened back in 1974, so it was quite a few years ago. I was quite ashamed of it initially. I wasn't about to tell people the story, that I had spent six months in solitary.

The thing is that I never did drugs as a teenager. I had a very sheltered upbringing. People would be toking, you know, smoking, they called them "spliffs" in those days, joints, whatever. I never did that. My drug of choice was always alcohol. I was quite happy with my Scotch, and I didn't think it was a good idea to mix.

For me, to be going to India as a drug mule was really out of character.

This happened through a fellow I met at a party. He seemed to be a really nice guy, and, of course, he was good looking, and I went home with him.

I guess I was a bit of a slut. [*Audrey laughs.*]

I saw the procedure, because one of the young drug mules, she couldn't have been, I don't know, eighteen or twenty years old, knocked on this fellow's door, just back from India. She had a suitcase, and she came in; this was early in the morning, I don't know, eight or nine o'clock. And I was there, in his apartment, which was quite grand, in Montréal. And he said, "If you just could excuse me"—something to that effect—"I just have a little business. I won't be long. Make yourself comfortable." And he handed me the paper.

I sat in a rocking chair in his living room, but I was not reading the paper, I was listening, and I thought, "Oh my God, look at *this*." You know, she had this suitcase with a hidden false bottom, and all the hash was in there, and he weighed it, and then gave her three thousand dollars.

And I thought, "Oh my God, this is much better than nursing." I think I was getting a little stale in my job and liked the excitement of the whole thing. I don't know where I came up with all that, but anyway, I thought it was a good way to make some quick cash.

We got caught on the first run—my friend, Peter, who was also a nurse, and me. Which was probably a blessing in disguise because while we were in India we had talked about doing a run of cocaine from Australia if this one had been successful. And we had no reason to believe it wouldn't be, because we were two older women. I was thirty-five and she was forty. Normally people that age were not drug mules, at least at that time. I don't know who's a drug mule anymore. We said that we would never haul heroin. Because that was really bad. But we wouldn't have minded doing some cocaine.

But it turned out that our bags were too heavy. They got greedy, that was the problem. They supplied us, at the Montréal end, with brand-new American Tourister luggage, a set of it. They said, "Don't have anything that's heavy. Don't add to the weight." I remember I had a nightie—that doesn't weigh anything—and very few clothes. And I bought stuff, in India. I had a few things made, like a sari, and I remember a long denim skirt that actually went into the suitcase.

But anybody picking those bags up empty would have said, "What the hell, is there a body in here?" We could hardly carry them! So that was a dead giveaway, as soon as we went to the airport. Somebody on the Indian side at the airport, handling luggage, must have alerted somebody in Holland.

Most of all, I felt really guilty, because my mother, who was a widow, was really affected by that, I think. The RCMP came pounding on her door at ten o'clock at night, here in Calgary. And my family knew *nothing* about what I was doing at the time, I had lied about it, of course. When we got caught, it was quite spectacular. It was on the CBC at home, coast to coast. I had cousins in Vancouver who heard it on the radio. And it was shameful, you know. My poor mother. She didn't know what to make of it. And here are the cops banging on her door.

They wanted to go through my stuff. I had shipped things to my mother's place, in Calgary, because I was moving there. And they did, they went through all my things. They were looking for my contacts in Montréal. They wanted the leader, but we wouldn't talk to them. They actually flew over to Holland and interviewed Peter and me separately. When I say "they," it was just one guy, and he had *no* personality.

"You tell us who's running this ship, in Montréal," he said. "Give us the name, and we'll spring you from prison."

We had probably only been in jail for a month or so, at that time. I guess some people would do just about anything to get out, but I knew it was a lie. We hadn't even been to court yet. How could the RCMP come over there and get us sprung?

And unbeknownst to me, because we couldn't collude, Peter and I, she didn't squeal either. I knew she wouldn't; I just knew she wouldn't. As for me, I just thought to myself, "I'm here now. I did the crime, I'll do the time," sort of thing. You know?

I was in solitary with a thick steel door, with a little window in it, and a curtain on the outside. When I say a window, it was a little pane of glass in that door, and they would pull the curtain that was over the window and look in, at any time, which is fine, rather than open the steel door. And there was no running water or anything. We had two buckets in the room, one with fresh water in it, and the other to use as a bathroom. Because they didn't come and get you. You couldn't knock on the door or ring a bell and call for help. You were stuck.

And with the steel doors, you couldn't see through bars, like in the movies. No, I couldn't see anything but this tiny little cubicle I was in. I could touch the walls with both my arms outstretched; it was really tiny. And the cot had a straw mattress on it and an old grey blanket. It was very primitive. It was *very* old, the jail. It was from the 1800s, and there had never been any renovations or anything. It was a horrible place.

There was a rat in my cell. It wasn't a pet rat or anything, it was this big brown rat. Well I was terrified, you know. It never came after me or anything though.

The communications happened when we went for a shower, because that's the only time I ever saw anybody else. We weren't even allowed out in the yard until after we went to court, which was three months in. I did start going to church there, because they took us to the chapel, this big chapel. And the women were all up in the choir loft. We never saw men, but you'd see them at church. Of course, we were crazy, and we thought, "Oh, at least we'll get to see some guys." It was just awful, when I think about it. [*Audrey laughs.*]

Anyway, I survived it, I don't know how, because I near drove myself crazy, thinking I was going to die in there. I lost so much weight. I mean, at the time, I was like, five foot nine, and I went down to 110 pounds in a very short period of time. The food was awful, it really was. But on canteen day, Thursdays, my order to the nurse would be for Mars bars or Snickers. Four bars for the week, and I'd get raisins, golden Sun-Maid raisins. The Mars bars and the raisins were what I lived on.

So anyway, it was quite an experience. And not a nice one, nothing to brag about. But between you and me, we had a fabulous trip.

I'm not sure it was worth six months in jail, it certainly wasn't, and there was a lot of humiliation along the way that you brought on yourself, you know.

But we were in a five-star hotel, right at the gates of India. And they weren't cheap with us, I'll tell you that. Money was flowing. Both of us went out and bought jewellery. I bought a beautiful diamond and sapphire ring, which, I forget how much it was worth now, but I remember having it appraised at Birks when I came home. I eventually gave it to my sister-in-law.

Anyway, we spent our money. We were only there a few days, so we asked for more money, and there would be money in the box for us, in an envelope. There was no shortage of money. So that was kind of nice. It was all first class.

Until we got to jail. [*Audrey laughs.*]

We were despised over there. The drug runners were absolutely despised. We were in there with, I remember, women that . . . one was an axe murderer. She hacked her husband's head off. Like violent, awful crimes. They were not looked down upon nearly as bad as us drug runners. We were the scum of the earth.

I had a lot of guilt over that stuff, you know. Because my mom was such a good, kind person. And she raised us right. I don't know what happened to Audrey. It was always Audrey.

It was very unlike me. I didn't do stuff like that. It wasn't that my parents were strict or anything, but I didn't go on a date until I was sixteen years old! I was dying to have dates, you know, like in the magazines. I read *Seventeen* magazine. Oh my God. I wasn't hard to look at. I wasn't a beauty either, but . . .

[*Ann: Well, I did hear a rumour that you knew Leonard Cohen, so you must have had a bit of game.*]

Oh yeah, I met him in Guadalajara, in the late sixties. Yes, I had a little fling with Leonard. He was a really nice man. I always really liked him. I loved his poetry and his music. But it was just a shot in the dark. I mean, that didn't last, obviously. I moved on, he moved on. I still listen to his music.

I've had a really good life.

The Holland experience was, you know, that was all my own fault, really, I couldn't blame it on anybody [*Audrey laughs*]. I took the chance. My brothers were all good guys, never did anything wrong in their lives. I don't know what happened to Audrey. But I kept things lively, I'll tell ya that!

Not on purpose.

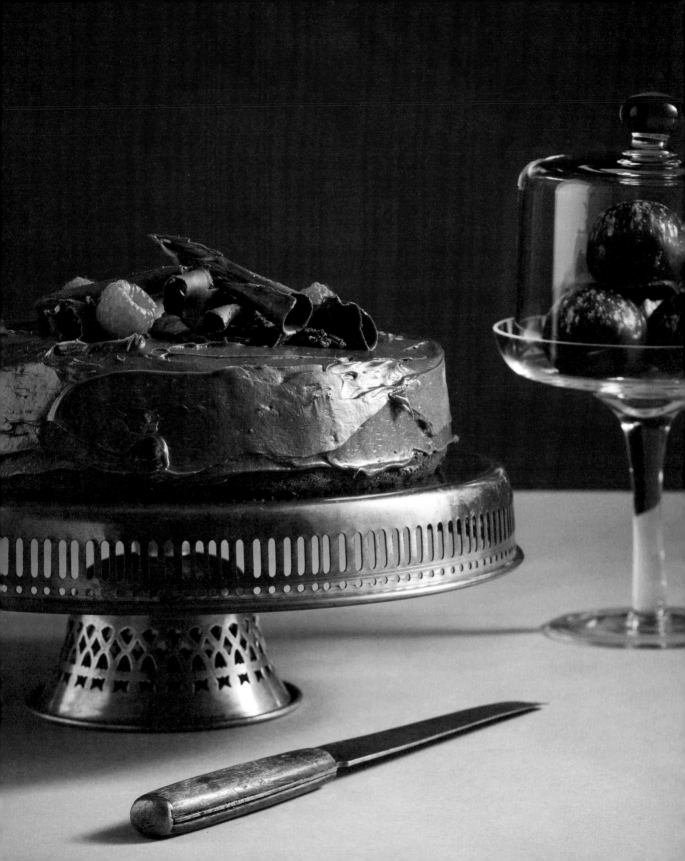

Raspberry Chocolate Celebration Cake and/or Double Chocolate Cake Pops

Yes, this is mostly a cookie book. But how can I leave you without being able to treat friends to a little infused cake for celebrations? This recipe will give you a wee 8-inch round cake—to be iced as per your favourite Pinterest genius, or as in my photo (easy yet beautiful)—or, the entire cake (or its infused leftovers) can be converted into these pretty double-chocolate cake pops. Making the pops will only result in one or two swears.

SUGGESTED MOOD/STRAIN

Let's go with *The Cake*, an indica-dominant strain that can help with chronic pain, insomnia, and stress.

If serving as 8 pieces of cake, 3 Tbsp cannabutter will yield almost 7 mg THC per piece.

If serving as 21 cake pops, dosing must be stronger per piece, so use 6 Tbsp cannabutter to yield about 5 mg THC per piece.

Cake and Cake Pops

2 Tbsp (for the cake pops; 29 g) or 5 Tbsp (for the cake; 71 g) unsalted regular butter, melted + butter for greasing the pan
6 Tbsp (for the cake pops; 85 g) or 3 Tbsp (for the cake; 43 g) cannabutter
¾ cup (150 g) granulated sugar
1 egg
1¼ cups (178 g) all-purpose flour
½ cup (43 g) cocoa powder
1 tsp baking soda
Dash of salt
1 cup coffee (can be warm or cold)

To make the cake or cake pops: Preheat oven to 350°F. Grease an 8-inch round cake pan with butter. Trace the bottom of the pan onto parchment paper, cut out the circle, and slap it onto the bottom of the pan. Cut a long strip of parchment wide enough for the height of the pan and stick the strip around the inner perimeter. And look, if you're just making pops, you only need crumbs anyway, so no need to stress about the cake sticking or looking pretty.

Melt the cannabutter in a double boiler or in a heat-proof bowl over a pot of simmering water. In the bowl of your favourite mixer, combine butters and sugar. Add in egg.

In a separate bowl, mix the dry ingredients together with a wooden spoon (flour, cocoa, baking soda, and salt).

Add the dry ingredients and coffee to the mixing bowl alternately in a few additions. Pour the batter into the prepared pan.

Bake the cake for about 25–30 minutes until it's springy to the touch and a tester comes away clean.

Let the cake cool in the pan for a few minutes, and then turn it out onto a rack, remove the parchment, and cool completely.

To finish the cake: This cake doesn't round much, but if it has, use a sharp knife to trim the top by scoring gently, turning the cake against the knife, and slicing the top off to be flat. Save that infused top for snacking on later (label it as infused, of course!). Flip the cake so that it's crumb-side down. Get creative with your favourite icing. Or, to top like the photo...

Finishing the Cake (option)

1 container store-bought chocolate icing

1 cup (170 g) dark chocolate, chopped

1 tsp shortening

Half-pint of raspberries

Finishing the Pops

½ cup store-bought chocolate icing

2 cups (320 g) candy melts or chocolate
   buttons

Oil

Edible gold dust (optional)

1. Transfer the cake to a square of cardboard covered in foil, so that it's easy to move about later. Slather the cake with your favourite store-bought icing using an offset spatula if you have one.

2. In that double boiler (or alternative), melt ¾ of the chocolate with 1 tsp shortening, until it's almost smooth, but not quite. Remove from heat, and stir in the remaining ¼ of the chocolate until all is smooth and melted.

3. Go watch one of the million "making chocolate curls" videos online. As the vids will tell you, pour the melted chocolate over a cold surface (like a clean stone countertop or the back of a cookie sheet) and smooth it with an offset spatula (non-technical name—icing smoother), thinner than you think it should be. Let it cool until it goes matte but isn't completely firm. Use your dough scraper to try to make curls. I suck at decorating, but even I got a few. Luckily, though, even little chips of bark look fantastic. Sprinkle the top of the cake with bark, curls, and raspberries.

To finish the cake pops: After you've baked and cooled your cake, tear your beautiful wee cake into pieces and pulse it into crumbs in a food processor. Add the icing, and the cake will come together as a "dough."

Roll little golf balls of dough, placing them on baking sheet(s) lined with wax paper or parchment. Refrigerate your balls for 30 minutes, and no more, until they firm up. (If you forget, let them warm on the counter to room temp so that they don't crack when you add the chocolate.)

Fill a mug ¾ full with candy melts or chocolate buttons. Warm in the microwave in 1-minute increments until liquidy, stirring each time. If the coating won't smooth, add the tiniest bit of neutral-tasting oil. Using a fork, submerge each ball in the mug, letting most of the coating drip off so that it doesn't pool below the balls. If you get cracks as the balls firm up, you can re-dip them. Put them back on the prepared baking sheet(s).

Refrigerate until your balls are solid, and sprinkle with edible gold dust if desired.

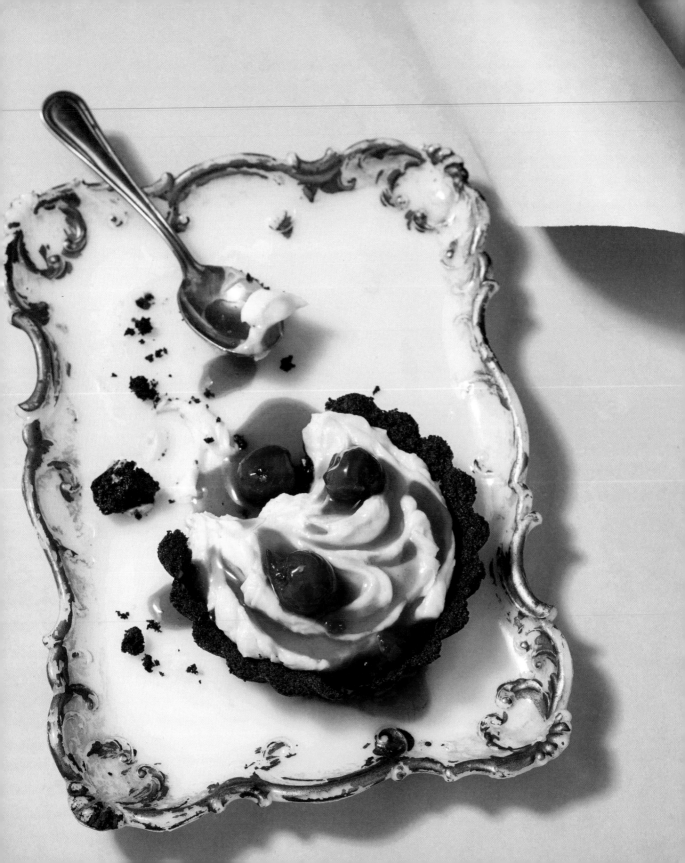

Black Forest Cheesecake Tarts

As easy as navigating the Black Forest.

Black Cherry OG is an indica descendant of *Granddaddy Purple* that combats insomnia and pain.

Makes 6 tarts with 2 Tbsp cannabutter (about 6 mg THC per piece).

Shells/Crust
Cooking spray
¼ cup (57 g) unsalted butter
2 Tbsp (29 g) cannabutter
20 Oreo-type cookies, pulsed in a food processor (or smashed in a zipper bag with a rolling pin) to make 1½ cups cookie crumbs, packed

Cherry Topping
1 jar (796 mL, 28 oz) sour cherries in light syrup—you'll use 2 cups of the cherries and 1 cup of the liquid
1 cup (200 g) granulated sugar
3 Tbsp cornstarch

Cheesecake Filling
About 1½ small containers (340 g) whipped cream cheese
½ cup (57 g) icing (powdered) sugar

To prep the shells and crust: Preheat oven to 350°F and apply cooking spray to 6 fluted 4-inch tart pans with removable bottoms.

Melt together the butters in a double boiler or in a heat-proof bowl over a pot of simmering water. Combine with the cookie crumbs.

Press the crumbs firmly into the tart pans and up the sides. Bake for about 6 minutes. Set the shells aside to cool completely.

To make the cherry topping and cheesecake filling: Meanwhile, in a small saucepan, heat 1 cup of the cherry syrup with 1 cup of sugar until it dissolves and begins to bubble. In a teeny dish, whisk the cornstarch with a little more syrup (or water). Pour this into the syrup and sugar mixture, and simmer until it bubbles and thickens. Add 2 cups of cherries. Allow filling to cool completely.

Meanwhile (again), with your favourite mixer, combine the whipped cream cheese with the powdered sugar. If you'll be piping the filling, set up the piping bag and a medium-sized round tip, facing it down into a glass and inside out.* Fill it with the sweetened cream cheese.

Carefully remove the shells from the little fluted pans by pushing the bottoms up. Jimmy (props to my Uncle Jimmy) a thin knife between each bottom plate and tart shell to remove. Pipe filling by starting around the perimeter of the crust, circling through to the middle. Or just use your icing spreader to fill each shell with a jaunty flourish of cream cheese.

Serve smothered in your beautiful cherry topping.

*If you don't want the filling to look rounded, an icing spreader, a.k.a. small offset spatula, will work instead.

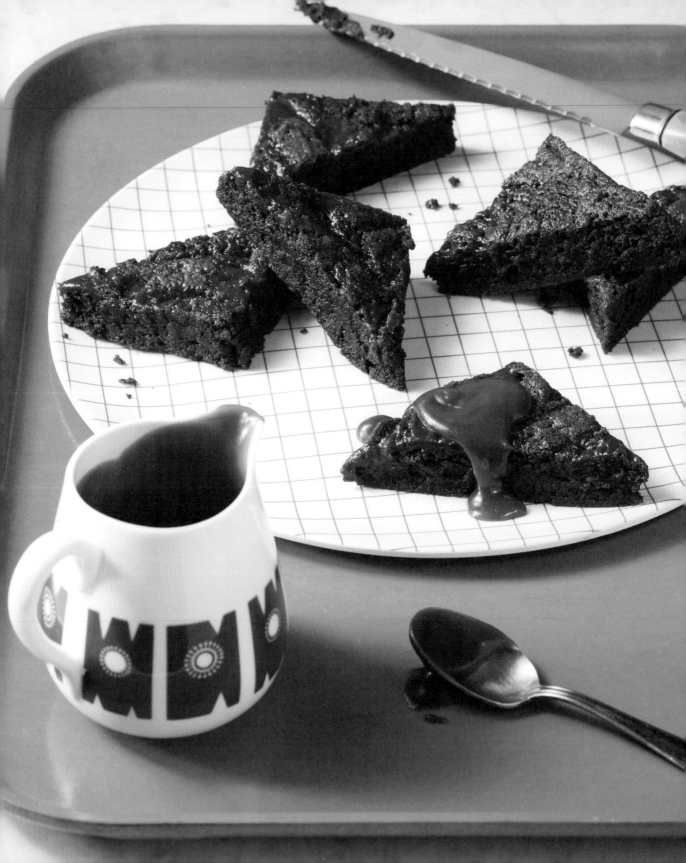

Caramel Brownies

Making this recipe is much easier than trying to eat just one of these brownies. But you must. No greening out! You can always substitute more butter in place of some of the cannabutter in your next batch and eat more.

Makes 16 brownies with ½ cup cannabutter (about 9 mg THC per piece).

Caramel Topping

1 cup (200 g) granulated sugar
6 Tbsp (85 g) unsalted butter
½ cup (125 mL) whipping (35%)
  cream

Brownies

4 oz (113 g) unsweetened chocolate, chopped
1 cup (170 g) milk chocolate chips
¼ cup (57 g) unsalted regular butter
½ cup (113 g) cannabutter
1 cup (200 g) granulated sugar
½ cup (100 g) brown sugar
2 eggs + 2 yolks
¾ cup (107 g) all-purpose flour
Dash of salt

To make the caramel topping: In a heavy-bottomed saucepan, melt the sugar with a splash of water, stirring regularly, over medium heat. Didn't know sugar would melt with heat? Now you know. The transformation feels very satisfying for some reason. Let it go just long enough that it becomes golden brown. (Don't burn it.)

Add the butter, stirring until it melts. Remove from heat.

Pour in the cream, give it a stir, and let your caramel cool on the counter until it won't roast the other stuff in your fridge. When it's all good, chill it to cold, for at least 45 minutes.

To make the brownies: Preheat the oven to 350°F. Grease an 8 × 8-inch* square baking pan, then line with parchment.

Simmer water under your double boiler or in a saucepan under your heat-proof bowl. Add the chocolates and stir in the butters. Add the sugars. Remove from the heat and cool.

Whisk in the eggs and yolks, one at a time. Add the flour and salt. Spoon the batter into your prepared brownie pan.

Dollop the top of the brownie batter with spoonfuls of caramel—you'll end up with about half of your caramel left over, which you'll reserve as sauce. Drag a knife through the caramel lumps to spread them a little.

Bake about 30 minutes, until a tester stuck into the middle comes away with bits of cooked brownie stuck to it. Let the brownies cool to warm on the counter, and then pop the pan into the fridge until everything is solid. Turn the brownie block onto the counter and peel away the parchment. Flip it and slice it into quarters and quarters again, warming the knife under hot water and wiping it between slices if needed. (16 pieces. In the photo, we got fancy and made triangles! You do you, just watch the dosing.) Serve with the reserved caramel sauce.

*For a 9 x 9 pan, increase ingredients by 25 percent.

Riley Cote

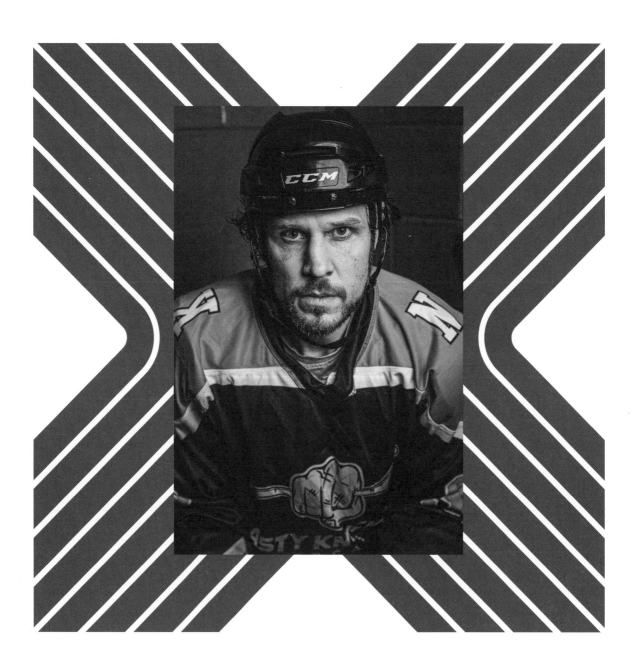

Riley Cote is an athlete and health advocate who co-founded BodyChek Wellness, a company that uses hemp and functional mushroom products to support physical and mental recovery. Riley played four seasons in the NHL for the Philadelphia Flyers, where he was known as an enforcer. Upon retirement, Riley founded the Hemp Heals Foundation, a non-profit organization that promotes cannabis as a renewable resource. He also co-founded Athletes for CARE, a non-profit organization supporting athletes in life after sport.

I was naturally attracted to hockey. I think that most Canadian kids are—Canadian boys, specifically. I grew up in Winnipeg, Manitoba, and my parents had season tickets to the Winnipeg Jets. Having that connection to the Jets, and kind of seeing it firsthand, I think that was probably really what injected the hockey spirit into me, because obviously my parents were fans of the game. My dad went as far as flooding a rink in our backyard, in the garden. So at four years old, I was playing half-ice hockey, and then from the ages of four, five, six, seven, I played with our local community club, Southdale. I eventually played Triple A, and then at sixteen years old, I moved away from home and got drafted into the Western Hockey League. I played with the WHL for four years.

In the Western Hockey League I wasn't an enforcer. I only fought twenty times or so in four years, so by no means was I known as an enforcer. But then when I wasn't drafted to the NHL after my eighteen-year-old year, I had to do a lot of soul-searching. It felt like the world was coming to an end, not getting drafted. But the way I'm wired, I just decided I had to find a way, to validate all the effort I'd been putting into this, and the money my parents had poured into it.

At twenty, I had the option of going back to play as a junior for an overage year playing other twenty-year-olds or turning pro. I looked at the guys getting called up to the NHL from the minor leagues, and it was guys with lots of points and lots of penalty minutes. My roommate at the time was drafted to the Florida Panthers; he was a tough guy, I had fought him before in practice, I knew that I could hold my own. But having one or two fights and holding your own thirty, thirty-five times a year is a different story.

I made the call. I mentally prepared to go into that next season, first-year pro, as a fighter.

I went to the Toronto Maple Leafs training camp, and my first shift in camp I ran Travis Green. Darcy Tucker came over, and Darcy Tucker is a tough guy, but he's not a big guy, he's not a heavyweight, by any means, so I wound up beating the pants off him, and, you know, that was the moment I kind of established myself as a fighter. I ended up signing with the St. John's Maple Leafs, landing in the Central Hockey League, where I fought, I believe, thirty-five times that first year, just fighting everyone and their brother. We won a championship, and then the next year I was in the East Coast Hockey League, with thirty fights. The next year I was in the American Hockey League, with thirty-five fights. And I kind of just worked my way up that way. It was all just mindset, really.

[Question from Ann that her hockey-loving relatives might not be proud of: Why the fights? What's the role of an enforcer in hockey?]

Using the physical body has always been a strategy in hockey. You can use your body to separate the man from the puck, whether it's with a body check or a good angle. Because when you're on defense, you're always trying to get the puck back and go on offense.

But outside of that simple strategy of just eliminating the man from the puck, as emotions start brewing and testosterone starts cycling, guys get pissed and cheap shots happen; crossing that line happens. And that's where the role of the physical enforcer comes in, in self-policing. It's observing an opponent taking a liberty on you or your teammates—usually your teammates, because, you know, you're a tough guy, so guys don't really take cheap shots on you—and you protect your teammates. It's accountability. You're the guy who's going to take care of business when shit hits the fan. It's an emotional game. Especially in the pro ranks, but even in junior. You've got grown men, grown young men, playing an elite sport, high pace, athletic, strong, and there's one puck on the ice and ten guys fighting for it. So naturally, things happen.

I played my NHL hockey career in Philly. And the Philadelphia Flyers won two Stanley Cups in the seventies as the Broad Street Bullies, right? Their strategy was being the tougher team. They had tougher guys, and the whole psychology of accountability, and of having to answer the bell. The Boston Bruins were kind of similar at the time—the way their teams were built. But eventually, everyone adopted that model. They all had two or three tough guys, and the playing field became somewhat even. So that Broad Street Bullies mentality didn't dissolve, it just spread itself around the league, versus just in one or two teams—tougher teams, bigger defencemen, that whole bit.

It's changed now, where there's still fighting in hockey, but the strategy of being the tougher team, like as far as having the Bob Probert, the Tie Domi—the tough guy that's going to be a difference maker—is really not part of the game anymore. It's more emotional fights, spontaneous fights, than self-policing.

Part of my story with cannabis was the decision to move on in my life, outside of playing hockey. You know, as far as self-preservation. It was like, "Okay, well, how much more can my body and brain take? Am I going to keep doing this and potentially be more crippled when all is said and done?" Talk about being accountable.

And mentally, being an enforcer is not the easiest role either. You're always fighting, and ready to engage in a fight. Sure, not every night is a fight, but I had to be prepared to fight every night. So there was this chronic state of anxiety, if you can imagine. There's no other way to explain it.

I'd seen the injuries that some guys have. They weren't just physically debilitating; there was also brain stuff. I had had knee surgeries, nose surgeries, finger surgeries, wrist surgery, eye surgery . . . And I was starting to feel old. My joints felt sore, and weathered, almost. I was twenty-eight years old in 2010. I didn't play a whole lot in my last year; we had a new coach come in, Peter Laviolette, and he didn't see the need for having a full-time enforcer on the team. He had won a Stanley Cup in Carolina without toughness, and he thought that he could come into Philly and do that.

I had another year with the Flyers on my contract but they didn't care. I was probably going to go down to the minors on a one-way contract, and I know how that goes. The minor leagues is a jungle. It's younger guys, full of piss and vinegar, trying to make a name for themselves, wanting to fight every night. And mentally, if I wasn't playing in the NHL, I didn't really want to fight anymore.

We lost to the Chicago Blackhawks in the final in 2010. I had this conversation with the General Manager, Paul Holmgren. He said, "I know where you're at mentally and physically. Listen, there's a job opening as assistant coach with the Flyers minor-league team, the Adirondack Phantoms."

I got off the phone call and thought, "This is it. I've got to retire. This is an opportunity to really give my body the healing it deserves, my mind, my spirit. And to really get out of this world of chronic anxiety." That was the exit strategy.

I had also just recovered from two surgeries using only cannabis for pain. So it was this whole sequence of events that was necessary for me to embark on this quest of holism.

I was introduced to weed at the age of fifteen and used it very recreationally. Throughout my junior and pro hockey career, I used cannabis intuitively, without knowing the depths of its medicine. I didn't know cannabis was medicine probably until 2010 when I retired. I knew that it was therapeutic, because it helped me sleep and to cope with the anxiety the night before a game. With those last surgeries that I mentioned, I just medicated with it based on intuition, based on experience, knowing about the opioid crisis, knowing that I was struggling with some substance abuse with alcohol and some other prescription drugs on the road, like sleeping pills and opiates and stuff like that. Knowing the dark path where that was leading me? So I just told myself, "I know I can manage these last two surgeries with cannabis." And I did. And that was when it was like, "Holy shit, this makes a ton of sense." It wasn't too far after that I read a book called *Hemp for Health* that outlined the entire cannabis plant as medicine. I read about THC, CBD, other cannabinoids, terpenes, and all the industrial applications.

I learned that patent 66300507 existed, where the U.S. government patented the antioxidant and neuroprotectant properties of CBD and other cannabinoids, and that prompted me to begin intentionally taking CBD-rich tinctures to help with the concussion-related effects I was dealing with. I also started taking psilocybin mushrooms and cleaning up my diet.

What also really grabbed me was the nutritional profile of the hemp seed. I was consuming a lot of protein powder, of course, from all this whey protein, animal-based dairy protein, casein, the whole bit; most people take whey protein and too much of it. And it's very gassy and bloating. I learned that the cannabis plant, hemp, hemp seeds, and hemp hearts were digestible proteins, full of omega-3 fatty acids. I began to realize that cannabis was this amazing resource.

It was no wonder that through those eleven years I had been so drawn toward cannabis because there's something spiritual that keeps bringing me back to it, with the therapy, sleep, calmness, and safe-haven feeling. But then there's also this whole other world of using cannabis, specifically CBD oil, for the brain. I had been in over 200 hockey fights, punched in the head over 2,000 times. So it made a ton of sense to start leaning on this as a legitimate regeneration and recovery tool for my brain.

When I retired, the first non-profit that I started was the Hemp Heals Foundation. Hemp Heals encourages using cannabis for all the things that I mentioned, but also for industrial and environmental uses—the fibres, building materials, food, and biofuel. I started the Hemp Heals Music Festival in Philly, and we raised money and brought awareness around the cannabis plant through music.

I began speaking more publicly around cannabis as a whole, and running into different athletes at conferences. We started advocating for true medicinal and recovery uses—regeneration, using the sports platform to normalize cannabis and helping to change sports policy. I co-founded another non-profit, Athletes for CARE. We provide a support system for athletes, as far as cannabis versus an opioid, and cannabis versus alcohol, helping transition guys after sport with the proper tools. We've also engaged in four or five different research initiatives with CBD and otherwise. It's not just selfishly for the athletes, it's using the experience we have, and the knowledge, and the networks, to do good, to build this out for the average person. Because there's an athlete in all of us. Whether you think you're an athlete or not, we all follow the same natural laws, right? We all sleep, and sleep is the spine of recovery. You sleep better, you perform better, and have less anxiety. You sleep better, you have less inflammation, you have less pain. All these things are connected. You regenerate. You feel better, you're more aware, more alert. It's really bringing out the athlete in everybody, and normalizing through sport.

That's how BodyChek got started. In 2014, that first Farm Bill in the U.S. came around that started to separate hemp-derived cannabinoids from marijuana cannabinoids. The Charlotte's Web story came out and these low-THC strains now qualified hemp under different laws so that products could be sold across state lines. [*Charlotte Figi, seven years old in 2014, had Dravet's Syndrome that resulted in debilitating seizures. The Stanley brothers, growers in Colorado, developed the low-THC strain Charlotte's Web for her that kept the seizures under control. Charlotte wasn't expected to live past age eight, but she beat the odds until 2020, when she sadly succumbed to a grand mal seizure that had returned due to other illness.*] BodyChek got into that space, essentially using marijuana genetics, but growing under the hemp laws to keep THC below 0.3 percent, and then selling premium CBD and functional mushroom products, which we're still doing.

We really just wanted to bring cannabis to the community that might not be cannabis users. Because thinking of cannabis users, lots of people think Cheech and Chong, right? But my mother is sixty-five years old, and she uses CBD tincture. She's a cannabis user. We try to break down the boxes of what cannabis is and what it isn't. There's a cannabis-based product for everybody, really, even if it's a topical.

What are my hopes for the future? At the end of the day, we're talking about Mother Nature. We're talking about an herb, an industrial resource, a goddamn plant. I mean, I would love to see it with way less legal red tape. It almost seems as though we're creating uranium and nuclear weapons or something, the way it's regulated.

I'd like to see this go like in Scandinavian countries and European countries, where you see CBD in almost everything. Like instead of pumping a vitamin gummy from some bullshit source, you're actually using a cannabinoid-rich tincture, and maybe that's in a gummy. But it's also important to understand the THC, right? There are probably far fewer people who respect alcohol as a substance, the way any substance is supposed to be respected. With alcohol, there's the mentality, "Let's go get drunk." But what happened to just having a glass of wine and actually respecting the alcohol? With cannabis you see a lot of the same stuff. You see a lot of extreme recreational users— and I do think all cannabis is therapeutic to some degree—but you can also overkill the nervous system, probably causing more adverse side effects than people think, as far as motivation goes and productivity goes. So raising some awareness around responsible, mindful cannabis use, I would love to see that.

I'd love to see more people able to grow cannabis plants in their backyards, just like growing a tomato plant. I'd also love to see people be able to apply for a Ma and Pa–type cannabis dispensary without having to go through the corporate model of showing $2 million in a bank account to even apply for it. Because again, you're talking about a natural herb—a natural resource.

And you know, in the sports world right now, guys are on their own to find their own cannabis products and CBD products. They're technically in the grey area because in the NHL they still drug test, although they don't enforce it where they're suspending guys for THC. I'd say that 90 percent of guys are using some sort of cannabis-based product, if not more. Obviously, you're never going to get to the point where guys are smoking weed in the locker room, I'm not suggesting that. But transdermal patches, topicals, massage oils, tinctures, and capsules can be really useful for recovery. Sports is nothing more than the work, the effort on the ice, in practice and games, that's the work, and then outside of the actual work, all the guys' focus is on recovery, right? We're recovering and regenerating so that the next time we perform and get to work, we're feeling the best we can, with less inflammation, less stiffness, less wear and tear. So I'd like to see protocols, by the strength conditioning and trainers, to get these guys on CBD. I'd like to see it where if a guy gets a bell rung, maybe he takes 200 milligrams of CBD to help minimize the effect of the concussion. It's a neuroprotectant, after all.

It's going to take some time. We're still talking major politics here.

One more thing I'd like to touch on is that there's something very spiritual around cannabis use. I don't think the spiritual topic is talked about nearly enough. Spirituality is believing in something bigger than yourself. That's intuition. That's part of spirituality, and just knowing. It's tapping back into Mother Nature, versus having no understanding of anything and just trusting someone's word for it. For ninety years, the government has told us that this plant is bad. They've been locking people away, leading to most people's idea of cannabis as a bad thing. Let's get back to what has kept people healthy for a long time.

It goes back to being based on a feeling. You're getting out of your head and into your heart. That's spirituality. Connecting back to source—source energy. Cannabis is that, mushrooms are that. Growing your own garden is that. That's connection. When you just smoke a joint with somebody, that's connection. We live in a world of just straight numbers and data. People are spiritually poor. When you lose the spirit of cannabis, it becomes 100 percent corporate Wall Street cannabis, and that's what most cannabis-culture people are fearing. It's going commercial, with leadership always trying to de-spirit people. Taking away things that give people power. Natural medicine interferes with their psychotherapies, and antidepressants, and anti-anxiety medications, keeping people enslaved to the system. But there is a huge movement.

The more people that bang the drum the better.

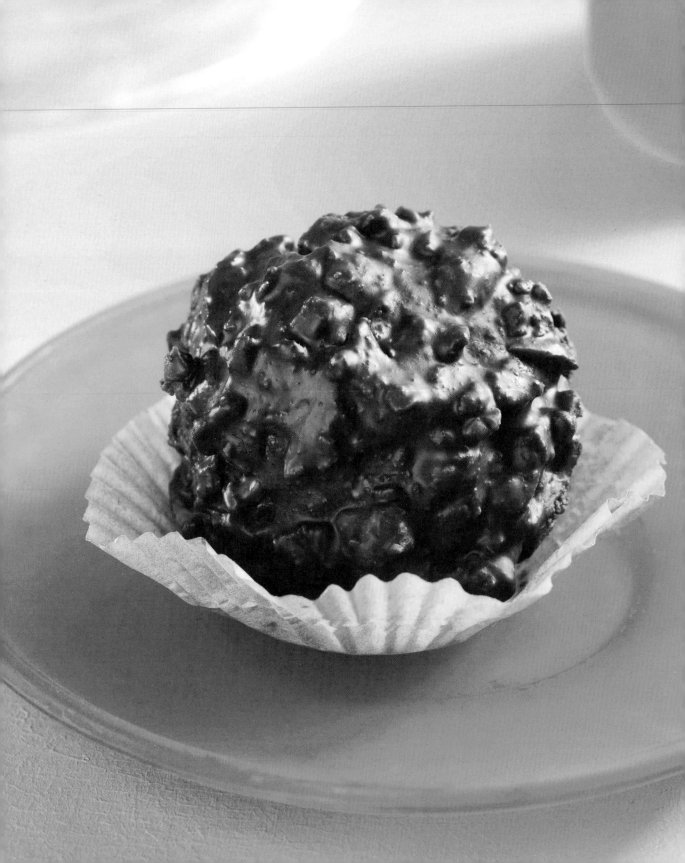

Mocha Hazelnut Truffles

I wanted to have at least one recipe for the java lovers out there.
This is it, and making it is easier than memorizing your most uptight friend's coffee
order. The coffee can be omitted to achieve a simpler truffle, if you must.

SUGGESTED MOOD/STRAIN

Caramel Kona Coffee Kush just
sounds delicious. It was born in
the Hawaiian Pakalōlō Seed Bank,
and unlike its caffeinated moniker,
it brings feelings of overall body
relaxation.

Makes 12 truffles with ¼ cup
cannabutter (about 6 mg THC
per piece).

Filling

2 cups (300 g) milk chocolate,
    chopped
¼ cup (57 g) cannabutter
2 Tbsp instant coffee
½ cup (125 mL) whipping
    (35%) cream

Coating

¾ cup (95 g) hazelnuts
Glug of olive oil
½ cup broken sugar cones
    (I used 2 regular-sized sugar cones,
    not the giant ones)
8 oz (227 g) semi-sweet chocolate,
    chopped
1 tsp coconut oil

To make the filling: Melt the milk chocolate together with the
cannabutter in a double boiler or in a heat-proof bowl over a pot
of simmering water. Whisk the instant coffee into the cream, and
then whisk that into the cannachocolate. Pour the whole thing
into a small bowl (so that the filling almost fills the bowl), let it
cool to room temperature, and then throw it into the freezer for
at least an hour.

When ready for the final prep, using a 1-Tbsp cookie scoop,
make generous balls of filling, rolling quickly into spheres with
your hands. This is messy. (Let the bowl warm a bit on the
counter if the filling is too frozen at first.) Plop the balls onto a
baking sheet lined with wax paper or a silicone mat and refrigerate
for at least a half hour.

To make the coating: Toss the hazelnuts in a bit of olive oil, throw
them onto a big plate, and microwave them in 1-minute intervals
until they're sizzly and fragrant. I like microwaving nuts better
than tanning them in the oven because I tend to burn oven nuts.
Don't judge.

With your food processor (or a big knife for the nuts and a
zipper bag/rolling pin for the sugar cones), pulse the hazelnuts
and cone bits together until fairly small, but not dust.

Break out that double boiler (or alternate) and get it going
again. Melt the chocolate with the coconut oil, and stir in the bits
of nuts/cones.

Dip the balls into the coating mix with a fork and place them
back onto the prepared baking sheet. Pop them into the fridge
one more time to chill.

Serve in pretty paper mini muffin cups.

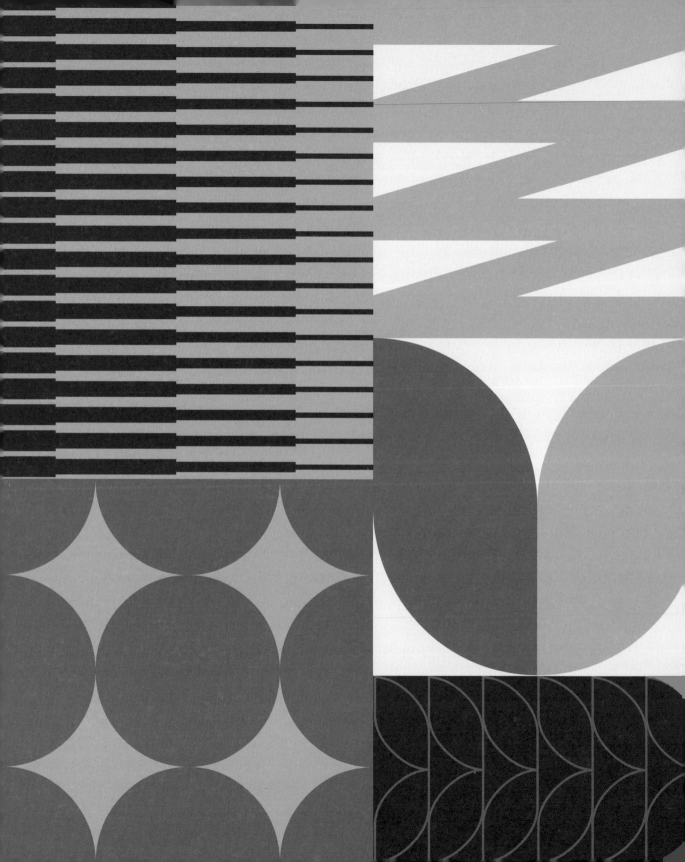

FRESH, FRUITY, AND FLORAL

RECIPES

STORIES

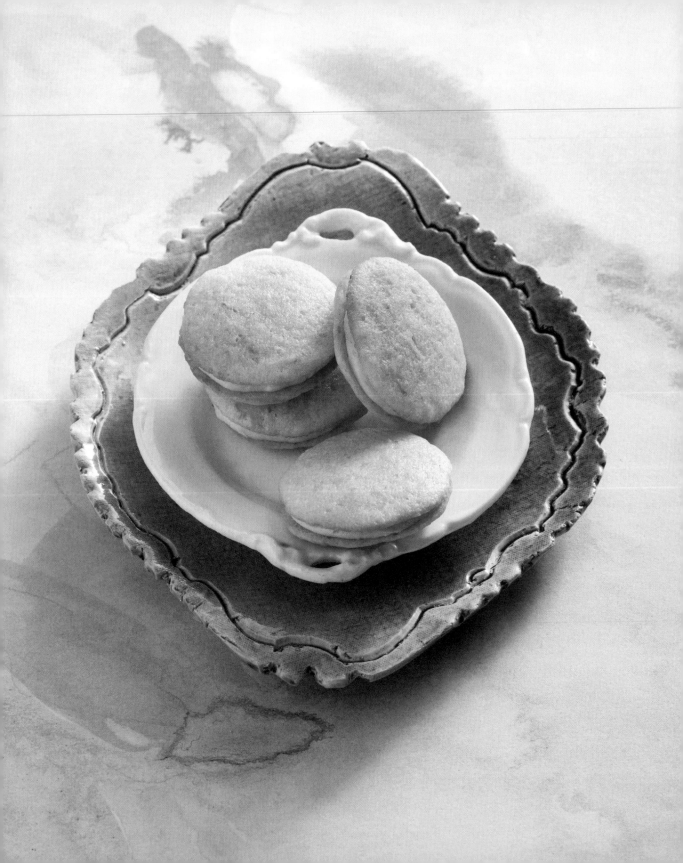

Lime Passion Fruit Sandwich Cookies

If you have a passion for piping things, this recipe is for you.

SUGGESTED MOOD/STRAIN

Passion Fruit is an energizing sativa that smells like a fruity drink on the beach.

Makes 18 cookies with ¼ cup +
1 Tbsp cannabutter (about 5 mg
THC per cookie).

Lime Wafer Cookies

¼ cup + 1 Tbsp (71 g) cannabutter
3 Tbsp (43 g) unsalted butter, melted
1¼ cups (250 g) granulated sugar
1 egg
Zest and juice from 2 limes (about
⅓ cup juice)
1½ cups (213 g) all-purpose flour
½ tsp baking soda
Dash of salt

Passion Fruit Filling

½ cup (113 grams) unsalted butter,
room temperature
2 cups (226 g) icing (powdered) sugar
3 Tbsp passion fruit syrup*
Orange food colouring

To make the cookies: Preheat oven to 350°F and prepare a baking sheet with a macaron mat.**

Melt the cannabutter in a double boiler or in a heat-proof bowl over a pot of simmering water.

With your favourite mixer, combine the butters and sugar. Add the egg, lime zest, and juice.

In a separate bowl, stir together the flour, baking soda, and salt. Add to the mixing bowl.

Fill two piping bags with cookie batter—you don't even need to bother with a tip here, just snip about ½ inch off the ends of the bags and roll with it. (Disposable bags are easiest because you can just fill a few rather than washing things out.) Pipe the inner circles onto the macaron mat with slightly mounded spirals of batter. As they bake, they'll spread to the outer circles.

Bake for 4 minutes, rotate the baking sheet, and bake for a further 4 minutes. The shells are done when they've lost their shine but haven't browned at the edges much. Let the wafers cool completely on the baking sheet before trying to remove them. (You can speed this up by lifting the mat and placing in the fridge.)

To make the passion fruit filling: Wash the mixing bowl and toss in the butter and powdered sugar. Start the mixer slowly to avoid a kitchen snowstorm, and then speed it up when the mixture starts to come together. Add the syrup and a few drops of orange food colouring.

Pair the wafer cookies so that sizes match, keeping flat sides together. This time, prepare one or two piping bags with filling (again, no tip is needed). Pipe filling in a spiral on the flat side of one of each of the paired wafers, and then "sandwich" the cookies together. (I guess this might be where the name comes from!)

*Passion fruit syrup is the star of this recipe. You should be able to find it wherever they sell snooty coffee or cocktail extras.

**If you don't have a macaron mat, you can sketch 1½-inch circles onto parchment paper for the same result. If you draw your own circles, don't pipe right to the edges.

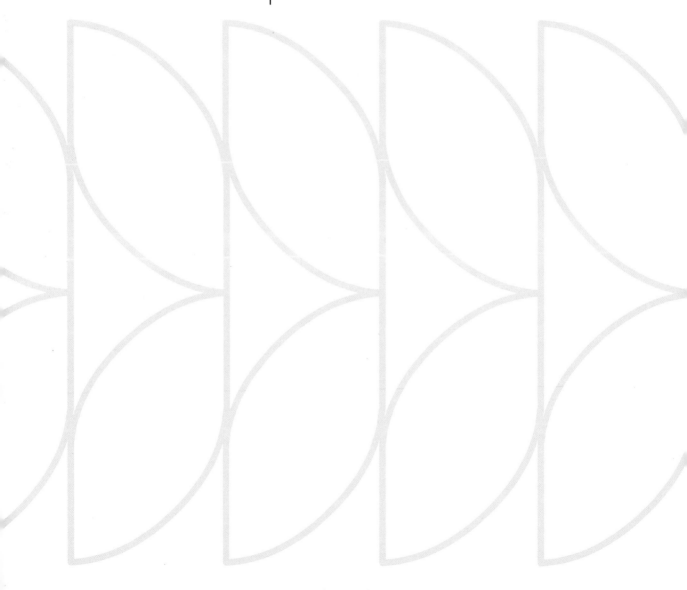

Lavender Sour Cream Cookies

This recipe is easier than telling the difference between lavender and mauve. I think that's all in the old-lady marketing. Which applies for either word. Maybe it's a 70- vs. 80-year-old thing? Please weigh in, old lady potheads.

I'm gonna be honest here. I thought this was a failed cookie. It was puffy, and I used a buttercream icing, which is kind of odd on a cookie instead of a cupcake. I brought a plate of them to some buddies and looked at my shoes. And they adored them. So, this is sort of a unique, smashed sour cream baked-donut-cupcake cookie. You think I was trained in France? This is the cannabis cookie school of hard knocks. Hence, it works. Enjoy!

SUGGESTED MOOD/STRAIN

Of course there's a lavender strain. *Lavender (Kush)* is an indica-dominant strain with dark purple highlights at the ends of its leaves.

Makes 38 cookies with ¾ cup cannabutter (almost 6 mg THC per piece).

Sour Cream Sugar Cookies

¾ cup cannabutter (171 g)

¼ cup (57 g) unsalted butter, room temperature

1 cup (200 g) granulated sugar, divided

1 tsp culinary lavender*

2 eggs

1 cup (250 mL) sour cream

1 tsp vanilla extract

3 cups (426 g) all-purpose flour

1 tsp baking powder

½ tsp baking soda

Dash of salt

To make sour cream sugar cookies: Preheat oven to 350°F and line baking sheet(s) with parchment paper or silicone mat(s).

Melt the cannabutter in a double boiler or in a heat-proof bowl over a pot of simmering water.

With your favourite mixer, combine butters and ¾ cup sugar.

Using a mortar and pestle (or food processor), grind reserved ¼ cup sugar with lavender. Add this herby sweetness to the mixing bowl. Add the eggs, sour cream, and vanilla.

In a separate bowl, combine the dry ingredients, using a wooden spoon. Add to the mixing bowl in a few additions.

Using a 1-Tbsp cookie scoop, drop lumps of dough onto the baking sheet(s), spaced a few inches apart (they won't spread too much). Bake about 10 minutes. When no longer shiny, remove from the oven. These cookies will look like dough lumps at first—depress them gently with a flat-bottomed glass. Use a spatula and transfer cookies to a wire rack, allowing them to cool completely.

To make the icing: In a small heavy saucepan, add 1 tsp lavender to milk and bring just to a gentle boil over medium-low heat, stirring occasionally. Strain, and allow the "infused" milk to cool. You're an infusing machine these days, non? You should wind up with a bit more than ¼ cup of lavender milk.

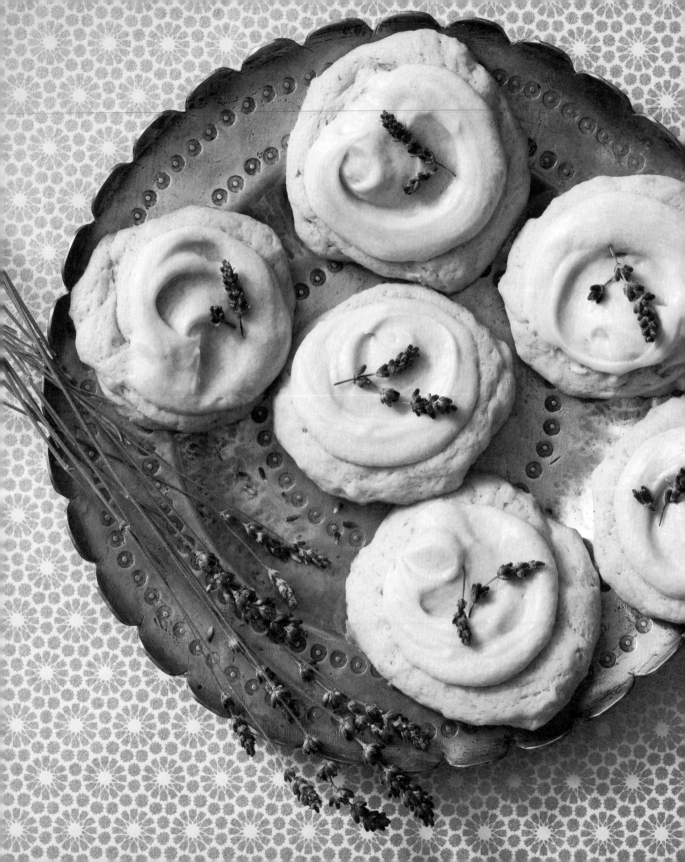

Icing

3 tsp culinary lavender, separated from
   stems and divided

½ cup (125 mL) milk

¾ cup (171 g) unsalted butter, room
   temperature

3 cups (339 g) icing (powdered) sugar

Dash of salt

Violet (or mauve) gel food colouring

Clean your mixing bowl of cookie dough, if you haven't already. Mix butter and sugar together, loosening with a bit of the infused milk here and there. In the end, add most of the remaining milk until you reach the consistency you like most. Add the salt.

Add violet food colouring, starting with a wee bit. (You can always go forward but never back! No pressure.) Stop when you've got the colour you like.

Spread the icing across the cooled cookies with a swirl, sprinkling with the reserved 2 tsp lavender.

*Culinary lavender can be purchased online, but I'm sure that if you find some grown organically in a friend's garden, it won't do you any harm. (Rinse off any shih poo pee-pee.)

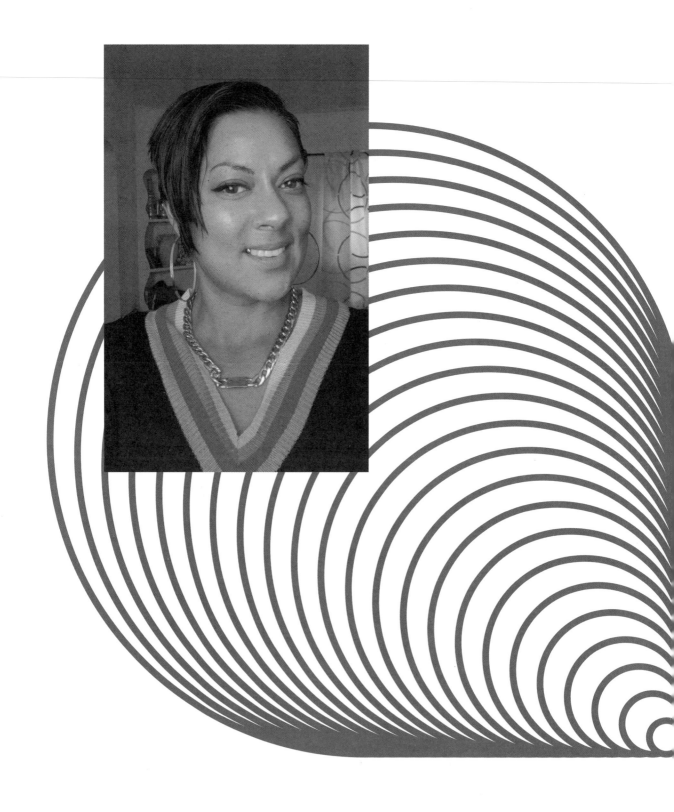

Reena Rampersad

Reena Rampersad is a fellow cannabis chef and Hamiltonian (although Hamilton is Reena's adopted home, whereas Stoney Creek, a satellite of Hamilton, was my childhood one). Reena has been in the restaurant industry for over ten years and owns the High Society Supper Club. She's a board member with four organizations, including the Afro Canadian Caribbean Association and the OrGanja Cannabis Society, and also volunteers with the Campaign for Cannabis Amnesty. Reena's restaurant recently fell victim to COVID's impact, so at the moment she caters (uninfused) events through rental kitchens, but she eventually wants to operate a cannabis consumption restaurant.

Yeah, so believe it or not, my first career was in social work. I worked with at-risk youth both here in Canada and in Detroit, Michigan. I saw a lot. My views on ganja and cannabis come from both my personal life, as someone who has always been around it, and in my professional life, in the psychology realm. I dealt with many families, and my job, of course, was to help put these families back together; to help them figure out what they needed to do to get their lives back on track.

Cannabis came up quite a bit, but if the household was completely dysfunctional, it usually had a long list of other chemicals and barbiturates tied to it. So cannabis, in my opinion, would have been the one that equalized it, and certainly didn't create the issues. It was really, really rare that a family would be in care simply because of that. It usually was alcohol or other drugs, or mental health, or other concerns. Not only was it not an issue, I recognized that it actually had healing potential in the realm of addiction and substance abuse.

My parents are from Trinidad. I'm of Caribbean heritage, so I grew up witnessing my grandmother smoking. I didn't really know *what* she was smoking, but I knew she was smoking. My father smoked. My mother never really smoked, I remember seeing her partake once in a blue moon. But I remember that the same thing that my grandmother used to smoke, she'd also make things out of it. She'd make teas. I remember once spraining my leg, and she took that same stuff, and put it with some oil, on the stove, and then they put it on my ankle that normally would have taken about five, six, seven days to heal up, but the soreness was miraculously non-existent by morning. So I remember that there was this thing that used to exist that was kind of wild. I never knew what it was until I got older.

I did observe, with my father partaking in it, that ganja was something that made him very peaceful and jovial. I noticed that he would laugh a lot and be very happy afterwards, which was a stark contrast from when they would drink. And my parents were drinkers. Unfortunately, that's ingrained in my culture—it's celebrated and encouraged. And folks were certainly different after having a bunch of drinks, in contrast to my dad's friends who smoked ganja.

When I was in social work, my father was experiencing some health concerns. The ignorance of society had somehow permeated me, and I had the belief that he was harming his body, so I did a lot of research. I went to Wayne State's medical library, which is one of the top medical schools in the United States, and I looked up every study I could that had the words ganja, marijuana, cannabis, or any derivative in it. It sounds like I did a tremendous amount of work, but this was done in a few weeks; there weren't many studies back then. I was expecting to find a bunch of ammunition and information to back me up, to tell my dad that he should probably limit his use. But it was just the contrary. I couldn't believe it. For cancer patients, I read about their experiences with improvement in increasing appetite, decreasing nausea, increasing their sense of well-being and outlook on life. I just kept reading more and more positives.

So that's where my educational background started up. But then maybe five-ish, ten-ish years later, I started to go through some personal things myself. I lost my father, and I went through a divorce.

I remember going to the doctor, not even for myself, just to deal with some matters with my dad's death. And the doctor said to me, "You seem really depressed. Would you like me to prescribe something for you?" He told me about a bunch of different medications that could probably help me and said I should just give them a try. I couldn't believe it. I didn't support drugs for depression for youth in social work, because I had seen those drugs make a lot of people worse rather than better, so I certainly didn't support them for myself. But I wondered if maybe I should think about trying something for my mood. I had discovered in going through my father's possessions—when people die, sadly, you have to do that whole duty of going through their stuff—I found a bunch of weed in my dad's freezer. I had put it aside, intending to gift it to his friends, maybe keep a tiny amount to have in commemoration of him or something. I wasn't really planning to smoke it. But I decided to roll one up.

Well, I'll never forget that smoke. Smoking weed for the first time as a youngster, and smoking it again as a mature adult who had a clue who she was and what she needed, were entirely different experiences, because older, I was looking for something entirely different. It didn't make me escape myself at all. Ganja put me much more in tune with who I was. And that finally made me recognize that all of this propaganda, and the stuff that they had pushed out in the media that I had started to believe, was just so false. I already had a mind of my own, but my eyes began to open to a lot of new things. I started to read more.

A few years later, I entered the restaurant industry. Pretty much as soon as I got into the kitchen, I started experimenting with ganja and ganja cooking. I already knew how to make butters and different things, but it turned out that all my staff were smokers. It really did make a difference for how the kitchen functioned. There were no flare-ups. There were no terrible attitudes. I started to experiment, and my staff willingly surrendered themselves as my guinea pigs. On their days off, I'd invite them to come for a free meal, and the meal would be medicated, and they would all tell me how much or how little they had felt it, and how they felt, most importantly.

One thing led to another, and I started making food in advance. I have a friend who's the owner of a vape lounge here, in Hamilton. He would have events, and the big draw of the event would be a medicated buffet, where we'd make munchie favourites, like ribs, mac and cheese, meatballs, fried donuts, things like that. I would infuse the sauces so that people could tweak their experiences. And we would never mix alcohol with the event. They were weed appreciation events, where connoisseurs or growers would come. They'd share their weed, there would be contests, like spliff rolling contests, or we'd watch a weed movie or whatever. I couldn't charge for the infusions, of course, which was fine, I did that as a method of promoting that this was a lifestyle choice that we should have. And it was something that I grew up with.

At the same time, I felt a burning urge to make people aware of the social injustices that had been done under the guise of prohibition. You know, the number of people who have been locked up or have lost their lives. And I'm someone who is directly related to some of the victims of the war on drugs. So when I speak, I don't just speak professionally, I speak personally. I've lost people.

My dad served jail time, more than once, for his choice to participate. The one time he was just smoking, and another time someone made an anonymous phone call and stated that he "had tons of weed on him." They came and did a search, and until there was an explanation, they put him behind bars for having his own personal amount. So that's my dad, constantly being accosted in society, with the shady looks he'd get from people, just for lighting up.

And then I had a younger brother who from a very young age started consuming cannabis. I believe he was about fourteen . . . maybe even younger than that when he had his first joint. Not really surprising in my culture, and not the most surprising among

young boys—you see lots of them smoking in the schoolyard. We have age-old movies and stories about all of that, right? So he started smoking from a very young age, but for a young melanated person, who identifies as being Black, and whose friends were Black, smoking weed can become a death sentence.

Very quickly, ganja got him a lot of unwarranted attention. A lot of ticketed offenses. Some nights in jail . . . and that continued to spiral. And when that ends up on your record as a young person, the next time you get stopped, and they see that you've been stopped before for it, they treat you differently. One thing led to another, years went by, traffic stops, they'd smell weed in the car, next thing you know, his car is impounded, he's behind bars, he loses his job because he can't show up for work . . . the list goes on and on.

It developed into an extreme anxiety. Police encounters? They never ended well for him. He'd been brutalized, too. He'd been knocked around by police; of course, that was never admitted. And so it got to the point where he would make extreme effort to avoid police. If he saw police or thought they were on one route, he'd rather drive twice the distance to work, or walk twice the distance to avoid them.

So one night, he got into an accident, and where most people would have waited for the police, unfortunately he had in his mind that this might have been his last encounter. Admittedly, my father had kind of planted that in his head as well. My dad, because of his experiences, told us that these encounters could end up deadly, and told us that we probably wouldn't make it home if we ended up engaging with police. "So don't be smoking weed, don't do this, don't do that." We had to be schooled every time we left home. I'm sure most people don't have to go through that, but we sure did.

So the night where my brother should have

felt comfortable enough to wait for police to come and help him, because he was in an accident, and genuinely they were probably coming to help him, his fear took over, and he left the scene of the accident. But he wasn't in any shape to leave. That was the night of an ice storm. A night where they said, "Do not travel." A night where things were freezing in seconds. And he left the vehicle barely dressed and without shoes on.

Long story short, he didn't make it very far. And I blame that on prohibition. I do.

[*Long silence*]

So if I can avoid other families having to deal with that . . .

I recognize that a lot of people can look at that situation and say that that was not directly related. No, he didn't have a joint in his hand and get shot by police. But I can tell you for sure, as someone who spent a minimum of ten years analyzing other people, and I was paid to do so, he absolutely ended up there because of prohibition. Had the attitude been different from the very beginning, when he was smoking weed as a youngster . . . If they had just told him to put it out, or maybe given him a ride home and told him you shouldn't be smoking as someone who's young, instead of putting him behind bars and making him feel like a criminal, and creating criminals out of good people?

Criminalizing people changes their minds. I know there are a bunch of "ifs" to it, but when I look at it, it's too long of a rap sheet based on cannabis fines and convictions to say it had no effect.

So that's that one.

And there are other people that I know of that have been shot straight up, by cops, because they've been pulled over because their car smells like weed. There's a friend in high school who we lost from a police encounter, and that's exactly what happened.

He and another friend were smoking weed and driving. And they were not speeding—they didn't make any mis-turns. It was a random police stop. And the smell of ganja elevated the incident, to the point where my friend got shot. And died.

And I'm sure that's happened thousands of times.

We want to prevent that from happening anymore.

If the world had been different—if things had always been legalized, and if the medical world had always revered it—I can guarantee that some of my family members would still be here.

We're getting there. I wish my dad was alive to see all this. It's pretty amazing, actually. I'm glad that we're moving where we are. Not quickly enough, by any means, and I definitely don't like the direction where a lot of legalization has gone, trying to really monopolize and corporatize something that should be available to many more people. But we're working on it.

It's a start.

Someone who is really brilliant, a criminal justice lawyer by the name of Annamaria Enenajor, decided to create the Campaign for Cannabis Amnesty, which is a non-profit organization representing those exact ideals and interests, believing that some of history's laws need to be righted, that awareness needs to be brought about, and that the government needs to create policies to reflect and correct some of those wrongdoings. I'm proud to say that we've certainly made some headway. We've created a lot of awareness. The government now is directly responding to our organization and our recommendations. They didn't respond the way that we wanted them to—we asked for expungements for all cannabis users, and they responded with expedited pardons or small expungements, which is okay, better than it was before, but it's still not much better for most people.

So you know, we're still going on that.

There are a lot of things left on my to-do list. Admittedly, I've been a little bit shy of the legal industry, just because I haven't been really satisfied with some of the rollout. But a lot of my friends from the legacy side of things have now joined the legal industry and are helping to create change from within, and it's really changing my mindset. And so for the first time I'm looking at the legal industry. I'm looking at potentially—not to jinx myself or anything—but I have folks who are interested in including my creations in the legal world.

I'm happy to be a part of something that's at least evolving.

So we'll see where that all goes. We'll see. For now, I'm over here, slinging dough, and literally flower, baking . . .

That's my life—circles under my eyes, working seven days a week. Hopefully, that will all ease up a little bit, and all of the fruits of my labour will start to bear.

I was lucky, very, very blessed, to be included in some of the early happenings of the industry. To be included as one of the first people to speak about many things, including food. But I'll always include the social justice side of things because that's what I'm most passionate about.

This is unlike any other industry. The folks who brought it and created it had it stolen out from under their feet, and then they were criminalized, and then they had it recalibrated and fed back to them, in a way that wasn't beneficial. And it's important that this story is told. I have no problem with what's going on right now, I'm so happy for it, because I don't have to look over my back anymore when I walk down the street and smoke. It's like wow. What a life-changing thing. I'm just really glad that society is finally catching up.

My final thoughts? I guess just for people to always have an open mind and speak out the truth. Yes. Speak the truth and have an open mind.

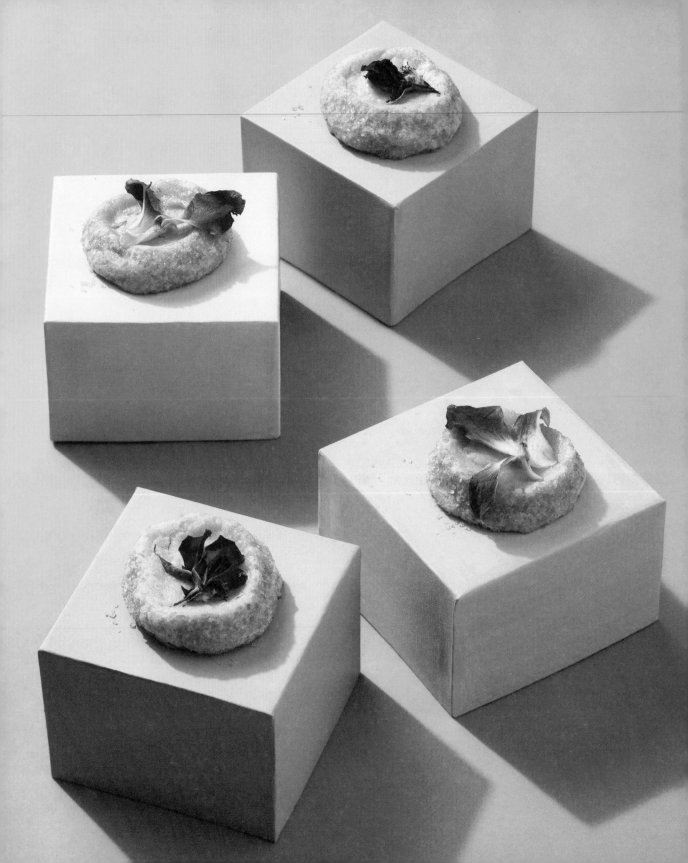

Shortbread Pamplemousse de Fleurs

This recipe is easier than picking a tulip from between your teeth.

SUGGESTED MOOD/STRAIN
Let's go with *Mud Bite*, for no reason other than it came up on Leafly under "Floral Strains," and I like the name. Apparently it was named for float houses in Alaska becoming mud locked when the tide went out. Indica-dominant.

Makes 28 cookies with ½ cup cannabutter (about 5 mg THC per piece).

½ cup (113 g) cannabutter
½ cup (113 g) butter, room
   temperature
1 cup (200 g) granulated sugar
1 grapefruit, zested and juiced
   (use all zest and about 2 tsp juice)
1 tsp vanilla extract
2 cups (284 g) all-purpose flour
½ cup turbinado (coarse) sugar
1 egg white
About ½ cup edible flowers*

Melt the cannabutter in a double boiler or in a heat-proof bowl over a pot of simmering water, then cool.

With your favourite mixer, combine butters with sugar. Add the grapefruit zest, juice, and vanilla. Slowly add the flour, and mix only until the dough comes together.

Roll the dough into a log, about 3 inches thick. Wrap in plastic wrap and refrigerate until solid, for at least an hour.

Preheat the oven to 350°F and line baking sheet(s) with parchment paper or silicone mat(s).

Prepare a plate of turbinado sugar and roll the dough log in it, pressing hard so that the sugar sticks. Slice the log into ¼-inch cookies. Space as many as you can about 1 inch apart on the baking sheet(s), returning any raw cookie dough to the fridge to bake in a later batch.

Using a pastry brush or small new paint brush, slather the cookies with egg white and arrange flowers toward the centre of each cookie. The flowers will dry and shrink, so in this case, more is more.

Bake about 13 minutes, checking near the end of the baking time. The cookies should not brown, so don't overbake. Repeat until all cookie dough has been decorated and baked.

Remove cookies from oven, and after a minute or so, use a spatula to remove to a wire rack, rearranging flowers if needed while the cookies are still hot (maybe with tweezers, depending on how "particular" you are).

*Edible flowers (a.k.a. fleurs): I get these from a fancy grocery store near me, but if you've got access to organic grow-your-owns, the following flowers are edible: marigolds, herbs of all sorts, apple blossoms, begonias, lavender, clover, impatiens, fuchsia, pansies, roses, small cannabis fan leaves . . . Go ahead and Google for more!

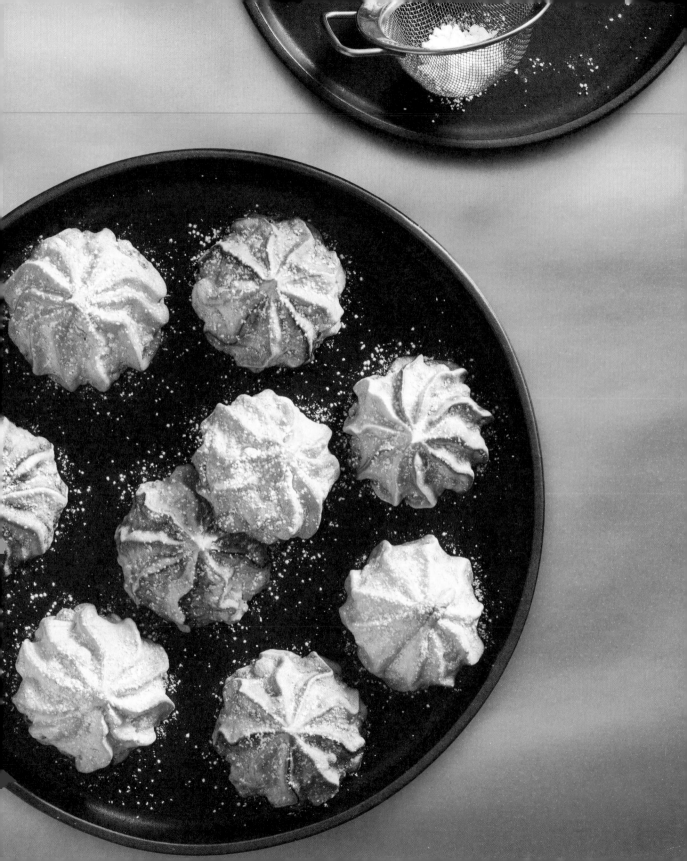

Lemon and Matcha Meringues

This recipe is easier than dancing the merengue.

SUGGESTED MOOD/STRAIN

Lemon Meringue is a good daytime strain that can encourage focus and energy.

Makes about 30 meringues with ½ cup cannasugar (only about 1 mg THC per cookie, assuming 3 mg/Tbsp; serve with tea or coffee sweetened with additional cannasugar to achieve dose). These treats are naturally gluten free.

Master Cookie

½ cup (100 g) granulated sugar
½ cup (100 g) cannasugar
4 room temperature egg whites
   (if your eggs are cold, let them sit
   in warm water for 5 or 10 minutes)
½ tsp cream of tartar

Matcha Meringues

Green gel colouring
½ tsp matcha powder*

Lemon Meringues

Yellow gel colouring
Finely grated zest of 1 lemon

So this is a lot of "mis en place" so that you can work quickly later. (I think that translates to *get your sh&t together*.) Line 2 baking sheets with parchment paper or silicone mats and preheat the oven to 300°F. Set up your piping bag with a tip. (I use the Wilton Star #849. If you can do this with multiple bags/tips at once, I'm jealous. Bring it.) Rest the bag in a tall, narrow glass, and flip it inside out, halfway over the rim of the glass. Set the gel colour(s) and a chopstick or new paint brush nearby.

Process your sugars together in the food processor until they become a fine dust. Give the bowl a shake, and keep processing. Repeat a few times. No one likes grit in their meringues.

Separate your eggs (toss the yolks or feed them to Sylvester Stallone), and add them to a clean, dry mixing bowl. Be sure not to get any yolk in there or your meringues won't work.

With a whisk attachment (or whisk), whip the egg whites until frothy. Sprinkle the cream of tartar over, and mix that a bit. Add the sugars little by little (like, spoonful by spoonful), fairly constantly and quickly, mixing after each addition until you get to "stiff peaks," which means the whites are shiny, and when you flip the whisk, the little cowlick is erect (guffaw).

Use the chopstick or paint brush to draw coloured stripes with the green gel colour up the side of the first piping bag. Remove half the whites into another bowl. Fold a little green gel colouring into one bowl and a little yellow gel colouring into the other bowl, being careful not to deflate the goodness. Fold the lemon zest into the yellow bowl and the matcha powder into the green bowl.

Use a silicone spatula to fill the green-striped bag with the matcha whites. Pipe prettily onto the prepared baking sheet, about 1½ inches apart, swirling around the outside and finishing with a flourish in the middle (they will gently spread).

Moving quickly, wash your piping setup, replace the bag if disposable, draw stripes with the yellow gel colouring up the sides of a new or washed piping bag, and fill the bag with the lemon egg whites. Pipe the yellow whites onto the other prepared baking sheet and pop both sheets into the oven.

Bake at 300°F for the first half hour, and then drop the temp to 250°F for the second half hour without opening the oven door. Let your pretty lil cookies cool and remove by firmly popping them off the sheet with a thin spatula or wide knife. The cannasugar makes these meringues look "rustic," which gave me temporary Tourette's at first, but then I decided they were cool.

Don't store these treats in the fridge—avoid humidity. Go wet-suit, or, at the very least, use an air-tight container. If they do get too chewy, reheat them at 200°F for 15 minutes.

Marvel that these light little cookies will bring even more lightness in about an hour.

*Matcha powder: Found in health food stores. This can be expensive and you only need a bit, so if you're unlikely to use it again, try to find it in small packets.

Alan Young

Alan Young is professor emeritus at Osgoode Hall Law School in Toronto. Professor Young spent his career arguing against intrusions of the state in the personal lives of Canadians by defending the accused and fighting for constitutional change regarding cannabis use, obscenity offenses, gambling charges, and sex work. He also co-founded and directed the Innocence Project at Osgoode, working to overturn wrongful convictions, and was awarded the Dianne Martin Medal for Social Justice through Law in 2018.

Before I forget, do you know about the famous Alice B. Toklas hash brownie recipe from the 1920s in Paris? Okay, because you're doing a cookbook, you should pay tribute to this. Remember, this is the professor in me coming out a little bit now. When Napoleon invaded Egypt, in the early nineteenth century, hashish was brought back to France. So in the *late* nineteenth century, there was a club called the Club des Hashischins, which is where a lot of famous writers like Baudelaire and Zola would go, and they'd try this little cookie green paste of hash and see how it affected them. A lot had very good experiences and wrote about it—except for Baudelaire, who wrote a famous book called *Artificial Paradises,* which is one of the only negative books historically about pot from a user. Long story short, Paris is always where writers congregated, so moving into the twentieth century,

hash was still kind of circulating, and Alice B. Toklas wrote a brownie recipe that was the first recipe ever written in the western world about hash. There were a lot of tributes to that in the sixties—Alice's hash brownie recipe.

This gets complicated, but it's interesting because of Alice B. Toklas. So I started doing this work in the early 1990s, but I wasn't going to challenge the pot laws yet, because the stigma was still too high. At the same time, I realized that one of the most important components to change in the law was changing information, and that it had to be a free flow of information, other than the negative government propaganda. So there was the law in the criminal code that prohibited publication of drug literature, which was any literature that advocated, glamorized, or promoted drug use. And it was a bit of a chill; even *High Times* couldn't circulate in stores.

It was around that time that I met Mark Emery, a bookstore owner in London, and I defended him on obscenity charges. We lost that case, but Mark was really into the whole dynamic of going to court and challenging the law, so I told him about the drug literature law; that we could challenge it. Lo and behold, Mark had a friend named David Lambert, who put together a guide of restaurants in London, Ontario, and, kind of as a joke, he put Alice B. Toklas's hash brownie recipe in as an insert in the guide, and the London police charged David with promoting drug literature.

So Mark and I ran to David's rescue. I prepared the whole constitutional challenge, but on the day we were supposed to argue it, they pulled the charge (because it was so silly). Fortunately, two years later, I was able to work on it again for the president of a group called NORML [*the National Organization for the Reform of Marijuana Laws*], which is a big group in the United States (in Canada, it's not as significant). But we struck out the drug literature law in 1993, and that's what resulted in this proliferation in Canada of grow books [*and magazines*]—Mark Emery's *Cannabis Culture, High Times*—and that really was, to me, the first turning of the page toward legalization.

So that was just a Mickey Mouse little case. It was an easy challenge, and so clearly a violation of protected speech. And even though people don't really know much about it, it really changed the marketplace of ideas, because everything until really the mid-1990s was simply one dimensional, one sided, and very negative. It was really like swimming upstream until some of the cases in the late nineties, when attitudes changed a bit. Oddly enough, I decided to challenge the pot laws in '97, largely because I saw that cultural shift. I saw it because I was an avid fan of *The Simpsons*. They started to make jokes about pot, you know, with Otto, and things like that. Prior to that, popular culture could only deal with cannabis on television if it was a negative story. It would be like *Melrose Place* or *Beverly Hills 90210*, and one of them would smoke a joint on an episode and they'd be in rehab in the next episode. So when I saw that slight cultural shift, coming out of the eighties' war on drugs, that things were loosening up, that's when I brought the challenges, in the late nineties.

The critical victory, though, was in Clay. [*Chris Clay owned a hemp shop and sold seedlings to an undercover police officer in 1995. Police also found small amounts of cannabis at his home. Alan and the team took his appeals to the Supreme Court.*] When I brought Clay, I knew it wouldn't be successful. The Charter wouldn't be used to strike down a piece of substantive legislation; they always defer to Parliament. But I used the occasion to get connected with media, as a communication exercise. We brought in seventeen experts from all around the world to talk about the benefits of cannabis, and also to talk about some of the risks, so that it would be a realistic and objective presentation, and it was covered in the media because they love pot. Journalists were the biggest pot smoking group I met through my journey. So we got great press, and then on the day of the decision, in August 1997, the *Globe and Mail* headline, taken right from the judgment, was, "Marijuana Is Relatively Harmless." Now, in the body of the article, they explained how the judge upheld the law, but when we talk about chipping away at this, that was in an incredibly significant national newspaper, and an old grey-haired establishment judge had scratched his head, wondering, "What the hell are we *doing* with this law, but I can't do anything about it," and that really propelled everything.

Even though I'd been reading vociferously all my life about cannabis, I was finally introduced to the medical aspect, which had been horribly suppressed, through Clay. I mean, I was a scholar, and it wasn't something I discovered easily; it was incredibly suppressed. But Chris Clay introduced me to two people who were medical users who he would supply to, and they told me their stories. They were very sick people, by the way. Lynn Harichy was an advocate in the early days, she had multiple sclerosis and died quite young, and Brenda Rochford had a neurological disorder. When I'd shake her hand, it felt like a bowl of Jell-O. These were very sick people, who said they

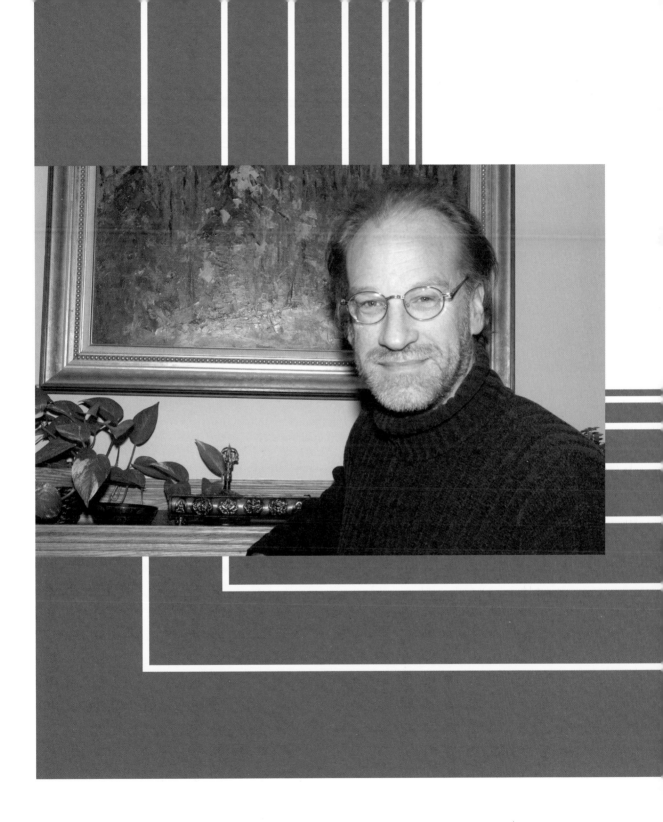

were basically living because of cannabis.

Anyway, I wasn't convinced that cannabis had medical use. I didn't know much about this. I just believed that cannabis was euphoric, and that feeling good when you're sick is just an absolute good. So I wasn't convinced, but I realized that the best way I could sell cannabis to the general public, who were still accusing me of trying to destroy the fabric of Canadian society, was to shift the focus a bit to medical use, because everybody gets sick, and everybody wants to be able to take the type of therapeutic actions they think work, and judges are largely older people who understand illness much better than young people and would understand that need for autonomous choice.

So I raised medical need in Clay, and brought in experts about it, and the judge decided not to do anything about it, saying, "Well, it's Chris Clay who's on trial and he's not a medical user."

But a couple of years later we were back in court with James Wakeford, a medical user living with HIV/AIDS, and an epileptic named Terry Parker, and ultimately, we were able to focus solely on the medical issue and get rulings that were the next big chip in the edifice falling apart—the biggest chip—because the government had to regulate and authorize medical use.

And to make a long story really short, marijuana just flooded the nation. Everything could be used under the guise of medical. The government couldn't control it—they lost the war. To use Mark Emery's expression, "We overgrew the government." Through the medical program, we had 40,000 people growing; the medical program fuelled what the government called the black market, which isn't so black, by the way, it's actually quite a pleasant market, other than some bikers that get involved.

And so the medical program really was the death knell in the law, because the government could no longer spend money trying to control cannabis when millions of Canadians were using it, and if you wanted to get immunity from the law, you just had to get a doctor to say you needed to sleep, or for whatever purpose. Now doctors were resistant, I'm idealizing the program, it was an enormous struggle with genuinely sick people, to get them marijuana for medical purposes. But by the same token, the whole medical program became the platform for just ripping apart the war on cannabis.

By the time legalization came around [*October 17, 2018*], I started to develop almost a chip on my shoulder because I had worked so hard on the human rights aspect of it, and I got a modest amount of money, but I did all of my work for free. Millions of dollars of work for free. So I mean, first of all, when legalization came, I was happy, because it was an achievement, and it was the right decision—an important public policy decision. But that day, two of the people from Clay came over to my apartment, and it was so nice to see them, by the way, twenty-five years earlier we worked so hard, all of us. But one of these people is a grower for one of the licensed producers, and because he got in at the ground level, no one had money, but they gave you shares. And anyone who got shares in those early days became rich, because it was a bubble, with the excitement of cannabis, and then it all levelled off. So here's this guy, these people I worked for, for free, twenty-five years ago, sacrificed a lot of time, a lot of my reputation, and they're talking about the millions of dollars from the shares. And I just kind of was waiting for someone to say, "Well, you know what, we should maybe pay you for your work." And so, when you asked me about legalization day, it was a bad day. But let me counterbalance it.

The next day, I'm outside, downtown. And it's the middle of the day, and I'm going to smoke a joint. And I was never really inhibited in terms of my pot use publicly because I always wanted to be charged. Like it would be an amazing thing for me to be able to convert that into a political battle, right? But I'm sitting outside smoking, and people are walking by, and then I realized something significant had changed. It's not only that I felt immune from the police, and "bring it on," I realized I was perfectly entitled to do what I was doing. And it was an incredible feeling of satisfaction. Because even though I never got messed up with the law, I protected people who got messed up with the law. You know, for a lot of people, pot is about parties, and music, and enjoying life. But for me, a big part of it was rescuing people who were caught up in the snares of the law for doing something that wasn't hurting anybody. It was like the world hadn't changed, but something significant had happened in my lifetime, that I had worked on. And it wasn't just a personal feeling of gratification because I worked on it. Often government doesn't get it right. This, they got right.

Unfortunately (there's an asterisk to it), I always did this really fighting more for decriminalization, which is the idea of just lifting the law. Not legalizing. Not creating an industry. I thought pot—to me, and I know it's a bit naïve—it's like growing roses, quite frankly, so I didn't see the need for any law. I just wanted people to be able to grow for themselves and not to have industry take over. And the reality is that we're talking three years later, and the legal market still only captures 40 to 60 percent, I don't recall what the most recent figures are, because having met with them many times, they weren't interested in my growers and dispensary owners, because they're into the idea of quantity and not quality, and that's a bit of

a problem. The few times that I've taken a foray into cannabis stores, I've not been impressed.

I guess my beef, my concern is, it's not pure legalization, because if you fall outside the contours of the legalized market, you fall back into criminal law. My thirty years of work were predicated on the idea that if something isn't harmful, it shouldn't be called criminal. In a way, you can almost say that the government chose to criminalize the competition, and I don't like that. But I'm not aware of a lot of people being charged. So I just don't know if it's a real issue, or just more one of political symbolism, which is still important. So that does bug me a bit.

The fact that people are making money off of pot? I don't care, that's the way the world goes round. In ten years, you're going to see there will be five companies, like Molson's, Coors . . . whatever. There won't be a lot of people doing this. It's very hard to make money doing it, and it's very complicated, but we're still in the frenzy period. The feeding frenzy.

Oh, and by the way, I will tell you this because I said, "Oh, I did all of this pro bono." One thing I will tell you on a cheerier note. [*Alan laughs.*] Do you know I have not paid for cannabis since 1998?

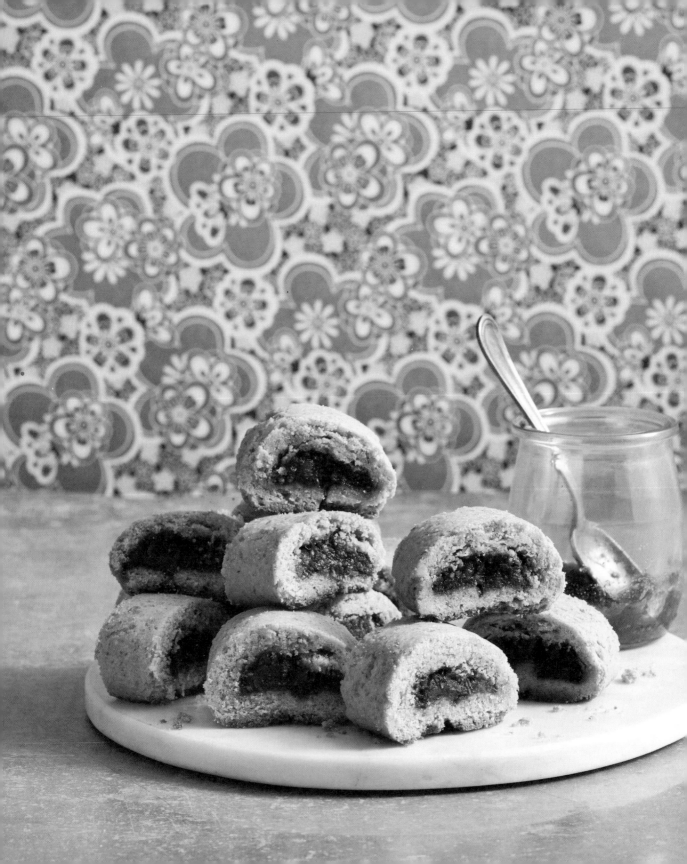

Spiced Orange Fig Newtons

This recipe is easier than knowing what figgy pudding is. The filling for these babies is adapted from Alice B. Toklas's "hash brownies," one of the first edibles recipes ever published, sent to her by a friend in Morocco. Oddly, Alice's recipe has always been called a "brownie" or "fudge," but it was more like a chewy spiced square and didn't contain any chocolate.

SUGGESTED MOOD/STRAIN

Alice is a sativa-dominant hybrid that encourages creativity and creates feelings of giddiness.

Makes 25 fig newtons with ½ cup cannabutter (almost 6 mg THC per cookie).

Dough

½ cup (113 g) cannabutter
¼ cup (50 g) brown sugar
1 egg
1 tsp vanilla extract
1 orange, zested and juiced (use all zest and about 1 Tbsp juice)
1¼ cups (178 g) all-purpose flour
¾ cup (117 g) whole wheat flour
½ tsp baking powder
Dash of salt

Filling

7 Tbsp (100 g) unsalted butter
½ cup (113 g) dried figs, halved, stems cut off
½ cup (113 g) dried pitted dates
1 Tbsp cinnamon
5 or 6 grinds of freshly ground pepper

To make the dough: Melt the cannabutter in a double boiler or in a heat-proof bowl over a pot of simmering water. With your favourite mixer, combine cannabutter and sugar. Add egg, vanilla, OJ, and zest.

In a separate bowl, mix the dry ingredients. Add the dry ingredients to the mixing bowl. If your dough isn't coming together, add a bit more OJ. If it seems too sticky/wet, add a bit more flour. Flatten the dough into a disk, wrap in plastic, and chill for at least an hour.

To fill and assemble the cookies: While your dough is chilling out, make the filling. Fill a kettle with water and bring to a boil. Throw all filling ingredients into a small saucepan. Add 1 cup of boiling water. Simmer on medium-low until your spicy Alice jam is thick, about 7 minutes. Use an immersion blender, if you're lucky enough to have one, to purée the mixture. If not, throw the spicy deliciousness into a food processor. If you don't have that, God bless.

When your dough has chilled, preheat oven to 350°F. Now here comes the part that intimidated me about fig newtons, but you can handle it. On parchment paper, measure and mark a rectangle that's 8 × 14 inches. Roll your dough to an even thickness to fit that rectangle. (If you keep it close to those dimensions, it will be the right thickness. You're welcome.) Use a pizza cutter or long knife to trim the dough into that rectangle exactly; when you slice bits off, slap them back around the edge to make use of all within the rectangle. Now use the cutter/knife to slice the dough in half lengthwise.

1 tsp coriander seeds, crushed with
    a mortar and pestle (or ½ tsp
    ground coriander)
¼ tsp ground nutmeg

Spoon a thick stripe of filling down the length of each long rectangle. You'll probably be left with a bit of extra filling, which can be used on toast tomorrow morning. Now roll your rectangle lengthwise over the filling using the parchment to help, pinching the long sides together, then flipping the seam to the bottom. Repeat with the other rectangle.

Put your figgy logs onto a baking sheet along with the parchment base and bake until just a little brown, about 25 minutes.

When the logs have cooled a little, slice into cookies about 1¼ inches wide with a sharp knife. Move to an airtight container while still warm—this will keep the cookies soft.

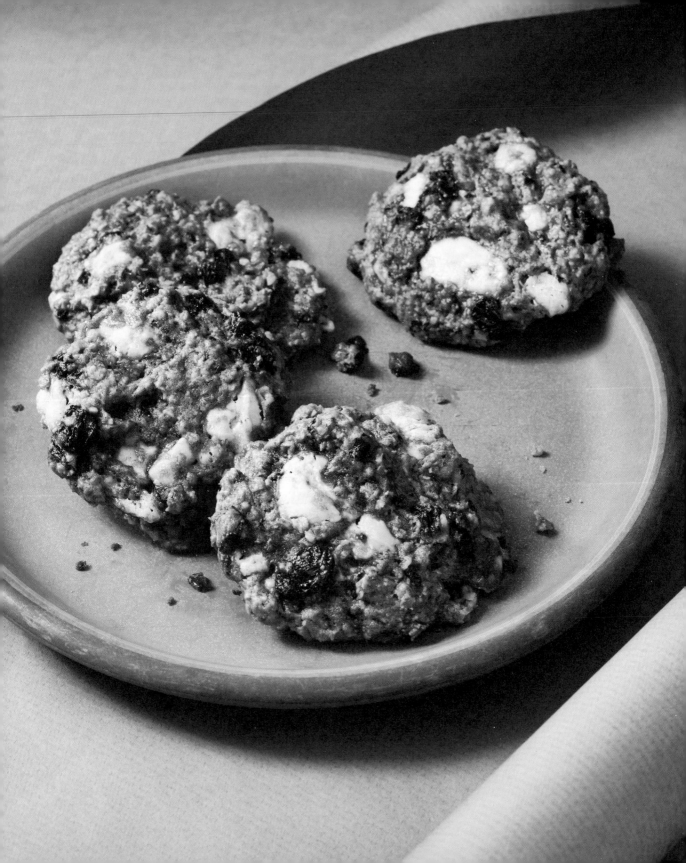

Violet Beauregarde Blueberry White Chocolate Cookies

Easier to make than winning gum-chewing championships, the Violet Beauregardes are kind of a cookie version of a blueberry muffin. Why didn't I just make an infused blueberry muffin? Go find an Oompa-Loompa and ask. I'll wait.

SUGGESTED MOOD/STRAIN

Blueberry won the 2000 Cannabis Cup for best indica.

Makes 30 cookies with ⅔ cup cannabutter (about 5 mg THC per cookie).

⅔ cup (151 g) cannabutter
⅓ cup (67 g) granulated sugar
½ cup (100 g) brown sugar
1 egg
2 cups blueberries (1 cup puréed + 1 cup whole)
1 cup (142 g) all-purpose flour
½ tsp baking powder
Dash of salt
1 cup (145 g) dried blueberries*
1 cup (160 g) white chocolate, chopped
2 cups (160 g) quick oats

Preheat oven to 350°F.

Melt the cannabutter in a double boiler or in a heat-proof bowl over a pot of simmering water.

With your favourite mixer, combine cannabutter with the sugars. Add the egg and blueberry purée.

In a separate bowl, stir together the flour, baking powder, and salt. Add to the mixing bowl.

Add the whole blueberries, dried blueberries, and white chocolate. Add the oats. Chill the dough in the fridge for at least half an hour. (This is important or your damn cookies will fall apart. Don't ask me how I know.)

Use a 1-Tbsp cookie scoop to glop generous dollops of dough onto baking sheets lined with parchment paper or silicone mats, spacing the cookies at least 1½ inches apart.

Bake for about 14 minutes until cookies are no longer shiny. Let them cool for about 10 minutes on the baking sheets before transferring to a rack to cool completely. (These are moist cookies and so are a bit delicate.)

*Dried blueberries: These can be a little tricky to find. My health food store delivered. (Figuratively. I still had to hump it there.)

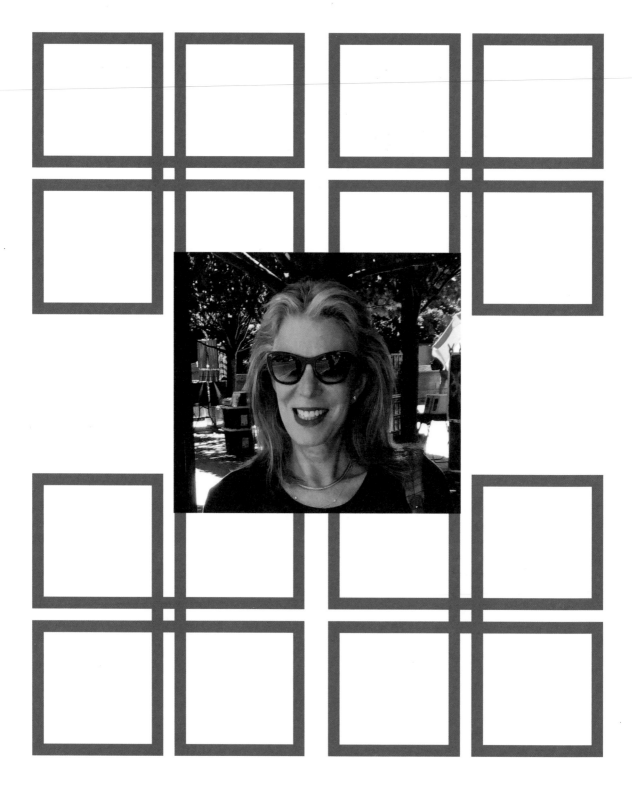

Louise Lipman

Louise Lipman has been a renowned art curator and publisher for over forty years. Louise spoke with me about how cannabis has helped her struggles with anxiety.

I'm not sure I have stories. I was thinking about that and I thought it's like saying, "Do you have stories about your antidepressant?" It doesn't read as storytelling for me. The stories of smoking and my own personal experience are internal. Because it's a solitary behaviour for me. Not social.

I'll give you a bit of history. I've always worked in the art-related world. When I was twenty-five, I was given a project to produce a book with twenty famous Canadian artists.

I went to Mira Godard, who [had] the "it" gallery at the time. She was representing Christopher Pratt, Alex Colville, and Jack Bush, lots of important Canadian artists who I needed to include in my book. And she said to me, "Why would any of them work for you? You're nobody."

Can you imagine?

I was twenty-five, and I *felt* like nobody. But that was very motivating, of course, as those things can be. I contacted the artists directly, and every one of them was generous and kind and wanted to be included in the book. That project kick-started what became a thriving poster business, and I moved to L.A. and started a successful gallery, so she did me a favour.

But I was alone. And I had to make it up as I went along. I'd wake up and have a complete anxiety attack: "How am I going to get through the day? What am I doing?" I felt like a fraud and needed to quell the anxiety and find the courage to pick up the phone and make cold calls to potential customers and artists. So I would have a puff in the morning. I didn't smoke to get stoned. I still don't. But I'd have a few puffs, and I found courage. I'd be able to do all of the things that had paralyzed me minutes before. I would be stuck, and I would become unstuck. I was able to go forth and conquer.

And I really did. *I did.* In fact, I came across some pictures of my other businesses recently, and the people and art were incredible. I was able to make the calls. I was able to talk to people, where otherwise I would have had it all in my head. So oddly enough, it's like an inverted social thing. I can't physically be with people, smoke, and socialize, but sometimes I can be alone and smoke, and then have a business meeting.

And the anxiety hasn't changed. It's always there; I have to manage my anxiety, and this is a way of management. I get more done. I stop ruminating and obsessing, get to my computer, do some work that's maybe been sitting on the back burner. You know, it helps to open the dam. And that's how I manage.

I don't smoke to get stoned. Just a little here or there. Like a slow drip.

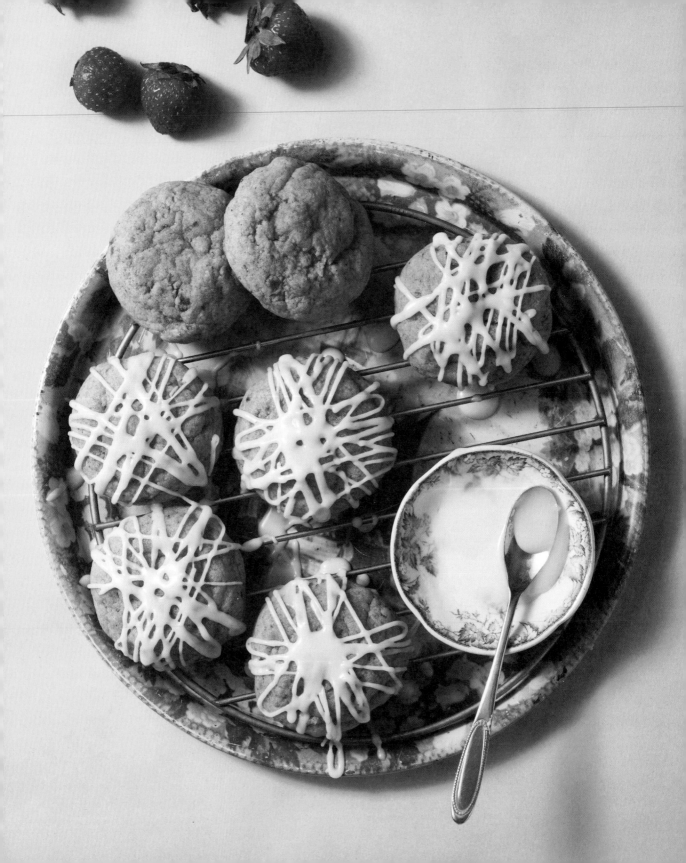

Strawberry Freckle Cookies

This recipe is easier than finding the heart of a strawberry.
I had a First Nations professor once who explained that the strawberry
is special as one of the first signs of spring, also sharing its heart-shaped
centre with you when you cut one in half.

SUGGESTED MOOD/STRAIN

Strawberry Amnesia is mostly a sativa and is aptly named. Leafly advises to "proceed with caution."

Makes 34 cookies with ½ cup cannabutter (about 4 mg THC per piece).

Cookies

½ cup (113 g) cannabutter
½ cup (113 g) unsalted regular butter, room temperature
1 cup (200 g) granulated sugar
2 eggs
2 tsp vanilla extract
2 cups (prior to crushing, about 55 g) dehydrated strawberries, divided*
2¾ cups (391 g) all-purpose flour
2 tsp baking powder
Dash of salt

Lemon Drizzle

About 3 Tbsp + 2 tsp lemon juice
1 cup (113 g) icing (powdered) sugar

Preheat oven to 350°F and line baking sheet(s) with parchment paper or silicone mat(s).

Melt the cannabutter in a double boiler or in a heat-proof bowl over a pot of simmering water.

With your favourite mixer, combine butters and sugar until fluffy. Add eggs, one at a time. Add vanilla.

Pulse half of the dehydrated strawberries with a food processor—this should get you about ⅓ cup of pink powder. In a medium bowl, combine this strawberry goodness with the flour, baking powder, and salt. Add to the mixing bowl in a few additions. With your fingers, gently squish the rest of the dehydrated strawberries in their original bag into small pieces. Stir into the cookie dough.

With a 1-Tbsp cookie scoop, spoon dough onto the baking sheet(s) (the cookies won't spread too much), rounding them into balls.

Bake for about 10 minutes.

Let the cookies cool for 5 or 10 minutes while mixing the drizzle. Use a whisk to add the lemon juice, little by little to the powdered sugar, until there's still motion but the glaze is fairly thick. Using a funnel, pour the glaze into a small squeeze bottle, and drizzle it over the cookies appetizingly.

*Dehydrated strawberries: These might be a little tricky to find, but the resulting flavour and gentle pink colour are worth it. Mine came in a "snack" brand from a health food store in 11 g packages (you'll need five), near the apple "chips" that mothers try to pass off to young kids as junk food.

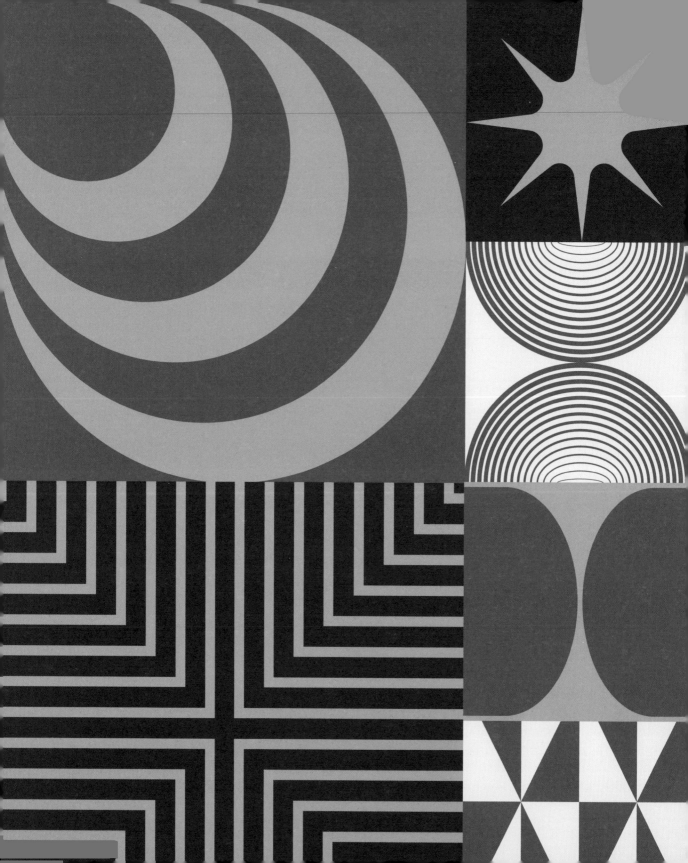

CULTURALLY COOL

RECIPES

STORIES

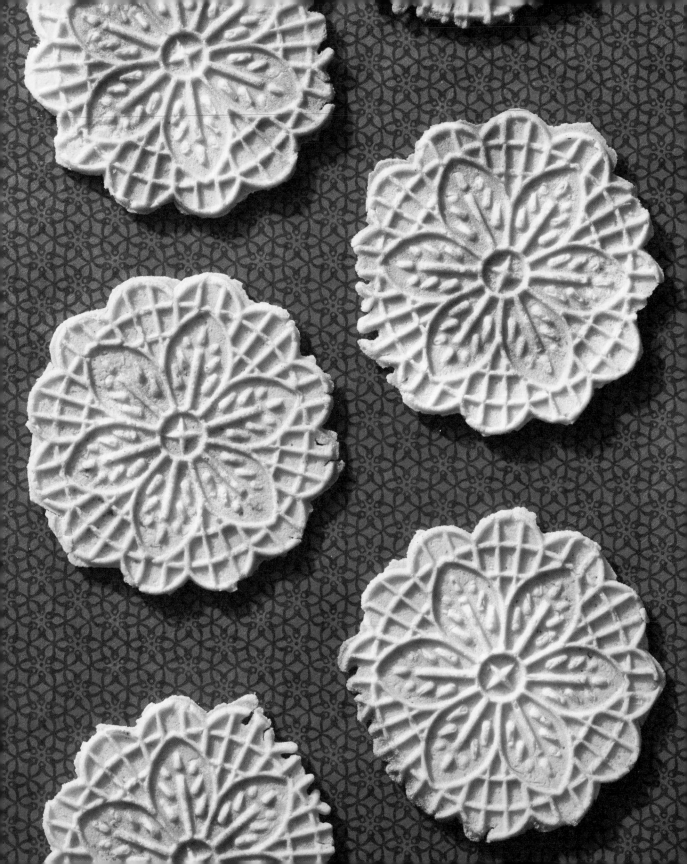

Pizzelle

This recipe is easier than saying "Pizzelle" in your best Italian accent.

SUGGESTED MOOD/STRAIN
Let's go with *Onda Calabra*, which translates from Italian to "Calabrian Wave," named for a popular song by Peppe Voltarelli.

Makes 20 pizzelle with ½ cup cannasugar (about 2 mg THC per piece, assuming that your pizzelles are 5 inches—eat at least two).

3 eggs
½ cup (100 g) cannasugar, powdered using a food processor
¼ cup (50 g) granulated sugar
½ cup (113 g) unsalted butter, melted and cooled
1 tsp anise extract*
Cooking spray
1½ cups (213 g) all-purpose flour
1½ tsp baking powder
Dash of salt

I shall choose to impersonate someone's cannabis-eating nonna with this recipe and prepare it by hand, using a whisk. If you'd rather be a lazy stoner nonno instead, go ahead and use the whisk attachment with your mixer. No matter the method, in a large bowl, combine the eggs and sugars, whisking for about 3 minutes, until the mixture is lighter yellow and has thickened. Add butter and anise extract.

Preheat your pizzelle maker** and spray it with cooking spray.

In a separate small bowl using a wooden spoon, combine the flour, baking powder, and salt. Add the dry ingredients to the mixing bowl in a few additions.

Drop spoonfuls of batter into the rear-centre of each pizzelle design (they'll squish forward). Mine took about 1 Tbsp of batter for each.

Close the iron and cook, according to package instructions (about 2 minutes).

Remove to a cooling rack with a spatula. Repeat until there's no batter left; you'll get great at making them by the time you get to the final one. Don't store in a plastic container or the pizzelle will go limp. Try a cookie tin or foil until ready to freeze, when you can wrap your pretties in plastic wrap and then foil.

*Anise extract: Star anise and anise are different, but either will work. If you don't like a gentle licorice taste or can't find it, substitute with vanilla extract.

**Pizzelle maker: Apologies for encouraging you to invest, but besides being able to impress with these pretty edibles, uninfused pizzelle will give payback in bake sales, holiday sweets, or feeding young people of any kind (substitute regular sugar for cannasugar, obvi).

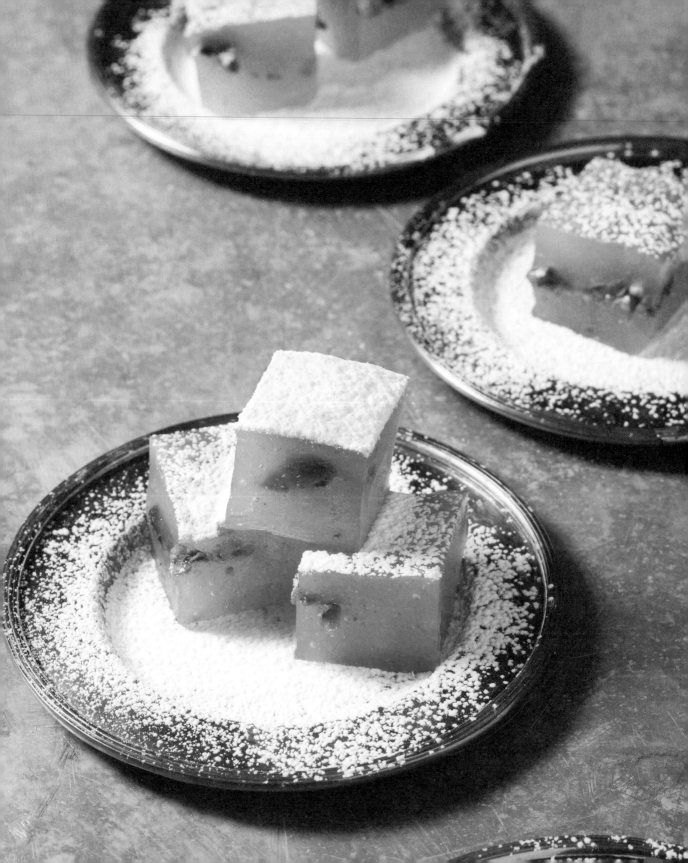

Turkish Delight

There's a reason Edmund narc'd on his siblings to a witch to get that magic Turkish delight. It takes some dedication to make, but it's so unique that I'm sure it will put all your friends under your spell.

SUGGESTED MOOD/STRAIN

The *Turkish* cannabis strain is an indica-leaning hybrid that is said to help to treat depression.

Makes 36 squares with 6 Tbsp cannasugar (only 1 mg THC per piece—eat 2 and serve with tea sweetened with an additional Tbsp cannasugar for a dose of about 4 mg).

Syrup
4 cups (400 g) granulated sugar
Slice of lemon

Paste
1¼ cups cornstarch, divided
1 tsp cream of tartar (white powder, stoners, not a liquid)

Finishing
A few drops of red food colouring
¼ tsp raspberry concentrate*
6 Tbsp (75 g) cannasugar, processed to a powder
⅔ cup (83 g) lightly salted, shelled pistachios, chopped
½ cup (56 grams) icing (powdered) sugar

To make the syrup: Combine the granulated sugar and lemon slice with 1½ cups water in a medium saucepan. Bring to a boil, stirring occasionally, and clip on a candy thermometer.

To make the paste: After the temperature has started climbing on the thermometer, get a second, slightly larger saucepan going with 1 cup of cornstarch, the cream of tartar, and 3 cups of water, over medium-high heat. Stir this until it reaches the consistency of thick glue.

Keep checking the syrup—it's ready when it reaches the "soft ball" stage, at a temperature of about 235°F. If you're a freewheeler who disses thermometers, you'll know the syrup is ready when you drop a bit into cold water and it stays together in a—wait for it—soft ball.

To finish the candy: When the syrup is ready, whisk it into the paste, a little at a time. Cook this magic for about 45 minutes at a low enough temp that it doesn't spit at you, stirring occasionally to keep it from burning the bottom of the pot. It will become a lovely golden colour.

Stir in the food colouring until the magic is a pretty pink. Add the raspberry concentrate and the cannasugar.

Pour half of the magic into an 8 × 8–inch** pan, oiled or buttered, and lined with parchment paper. (Trace the pan onto parchment, cut it out, and stick it to the bottom of the oiled or buttered pan.) Sprinkle with the chopped pistachios. Top with the remaining magic jelly batter.

Chill overnight until firm.

Slice around the edge of the delight with a sharp, thin knife, to help with the release from the pan. Mix together the icing sugar and the remaining ¼ cup cornstarch in a small bowl, and then dust a flat work surface with it. Turn the Turkish delight onto the surface. Using a pizza cutter or big sharp knife, slice the Turkish delight into 6 strips. Slice each strip into 6 squares. Toss the delightful cubes in the mixture of powdered sugar and cornstarch. Tap off the excess, and you've nailed it!

*Raspberry concentrate: I used a bottle by LorAnn Gourmet for this recipe, which says "four times as strong as extracts." If you can't find concentrate, use extract and increase to 1 tsp.

**Increase ingredient amounts by one quarter if you're using a 9 × 9–inch pan.

Chris Martin

I serendipitously "met" Chris Martin online when he followed my Facebook page. When I get a new follower I tend to creep them a little, to learn more about who has connected. Turned out that with Chris, rather than me flipping through photos of kids, dogs, and political views, he had an entire documentary about his life and experience as someone who had gone to prison for working in the cannabis space as a bit of an early adopter; he had been facing 130 years in prison for multiple non-violent cannabis-related felonies. I had been looking to interview someone who had paid a high price for something I take for granted—sharing weed with people who enjoy or need it—so Chris came along at exactly the right time. Chris had already told more of his story than I could ever ask in his documentary, *Haters Make Me Famous*, so rather than interviewing him, I decided to take snippets directly from his movie and present them to you below. I've added some transitions/explanations to help with flow. Chris and I are in touch, and he's been very gracious with supporting this book. I can't go into every detail of Chris's story (I'll probably get my hand slapped by an editor for the length of this piece already), but I encourage you to watch his whole film; you can find it on Amazon Prime in the U.S., or on Tubi here in Canada and elsewhere.

A few messages affected me strongly with Chris's story. One: whoever you are, you can be a mentor to someone and make a world of difference. (I didn't have much space to highlight these people, but Chris had them, and he was stronger for it. Watch the film.) And a little true love doesn't hurt anybody, if you're lucky enough to find it. Also, whatever cards you're dealt, you're capable of overcoming obstacles and becoming a great person; but if you do meet someone with a shitty hand, help them improve their cards (see Point #1). And finally, it might be tempting to judge someone like Chris for dealing pot in an illegal marketplace, but if you were/are using even a little pot in that kind of environment, remember that there has always been someone taking great risks for you, as an early-adoption entrepreneur, behind the scenes. Be kind with your consideration, and support the Weldon Project, Mission Green, and organizations like them.

Chris: From the beginning, it was pretty rough. I was born in Virginia in 1975. My parents were pretty young. They split before I really remember anything. My stepdad, Max, came into the picture then. They met, and put me in a backpack, and we would travel across the country where we ended up in Topeka, Kansas.

Nine years old was when the troubles started. My stepdad was a drinker, my mom was a drug addict, and that was a terrible combo. My role in the family as oldest was either to defend my mom, or don't. Defend the children. Well, I ended up taking on both roles, because . . . it's human? It's what we do? As I'd defend my mom, it was tag team. Stepdad would jump in, and, "Oh, you want to get in our business?" Or Mom would turn that role. So I tried to avoid that situation just by taking care of the kids. I'm the oldest of eight. The physical side—I was kind of the warrior on that. I took most of that.

I learned really quickly that I didn't want to get hit by either one of them, so I ran away.

[*When I was thirteen*] my mom . . . was running a bar. [*Through the bar*] she met a guy named Mike. And Mike was "our hero." He came to "save us," from the beatings, and the violence. But in all actuality, he became the worst offender of both. My stepdad Mike hit my mom with a full beer. Knocked her unconscious, broke her fingers with his hands, and when she came to, she got grabbed by the throat and picked up. I snuck into the kitchen, grabbed a knife, and I stabbed him. It was the only way I could get him off of her.

[*Chris jumped out of a second-story window and ran to a friend's house. The police photographed his many injuries, including bite marks. Although Chris had run away and returned home time and again, feeling responsibility toward his brothers and sisters, this time was different.*]

I had to choose the lesser of two evils. You know you're going to get beat up at Mom's. You run your odds at the group home.

An attempted rape happened, and I learned how to defend myself at a very young age. The first time I ever fought for my life was at the emergency shelter. It's pretty bad when you're less afraid to live on the street than you are to live in a boys' home, in a shelter, or in your own house. I was willing to risk it. I went through a total of forty-two placements from the time I was nine to the time I was eighteen. I went to eight different high schools.

I finally turned eighteen. I was kicked out of the system. Next thing you know, I end up in Prescott, Arizona, in a snowstorm, pitching an eight-pitch tryout for Yavapai Community College. I felt like life had finally made a change in direction for me. Three months later, I was in prison for cannabis. Didn't see that one coming.

It was pretty crazy for me to land at Yavapai, when I got recruited. Because coming from Topeka, where it's very ghetto and very bad neighbourhoods, you live your life that way, in foster homes and group homes, and then you come to white suburbia, Prescott, Arizona, living in a dorm, with a bunch of rich kids, who have no idea the struggle or the life that we lived or went through.

Not having a family to support you while you're in college is a tough deal. I thought I could do it on my own, and I had no money! I had no job, I had no way to even buy shoes. A couple of months in I had to find a way to take care of myself, and coming from the streets, and coming from my background, it was back to the drug scene. So I met a guy that had some weed, and the rest was history. I got caught with a joint in my dorm room. They raided my dorm thinking I was selling pot, which I was, but they didn't pull the mirror out and check the drywall for the eleven pounds I had hidden. They actually found the one personal joint I had in the top drawer, and I got three years for it. I got charged with possession of a dangerous drug in a drug-free school zone, and they gave me three years because the judge saw I grew up in group homes.

Lost my scholarship, never got to play one game on the field, and that was the end of my tenure at Yavapai College.

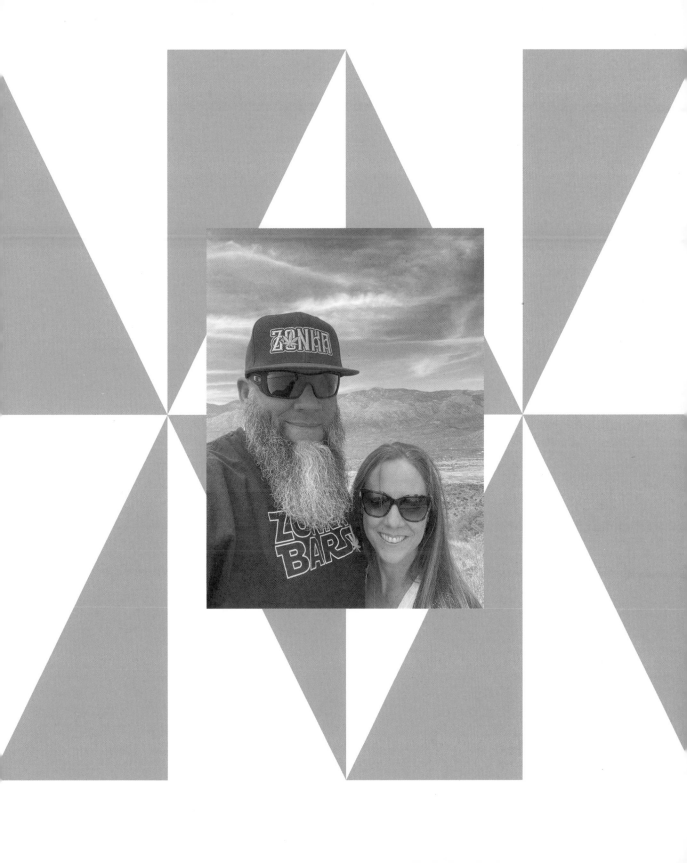

The first time I saw Andi, I knew she was the one. In all seriousness, I've known since that day, and every day since then. She'll tell you—every time she would come around, even if it had been two years, I would drop everything I was doing . . . any*one*, I was doing. Literally. I would leave them where they were, and I would go pick her up, or I would go see her. I just had to convince *her* that she was the one.

I was the president of the Desert Eagles Motorcycle Club. I was a member of the club for almost three years. I worked my rank from prospect to president in a matter of under a year. That happened mainly because of who I am. I mean, one, I'm a no-bullshit guy. I know how to run a program of brothers. We really took pride in [*the*] clubhouse. We utilized this not only for us but for business purposes and for our families. This gave us a great way for us to have a location to go hang out, in the back area; we had a "dunk a prospect" tank, we did Olympics for the kids, spoon races, water balloon fights, concerts, MS runs, cancer fundraisers, you name it. Anything we could do publicly here, we did it.

Andi: So when Chris first joined the motorcycle club, I was nervous. Chris was raised with it—his dad was into them. I didn't know too much besides what you see on TV, which is Hollywood, they shoot people, they're mean, they're not nice to women, you know, all the stuff you see and hear. So that was my first thing, was "oh no," but he made sure that it [*was*] a family club. We want[*ed*] to do right in the community and show that we [*were*] trying to be different than what people automatically think. It was a newer club, so I knew, like, "they need him," they see who he is and how he is. I think they all knew that, too—he's just a leader. You can just tell. That's who he is. He's a leader.

Chris: Then, in 2007 I was diagnosed with Crohn's. I had always medicated with cannabis and not realized that's what I was doing. I knew it made me feel better, I knew that when I ate it my stomach responded, but I didn't put two and two together as medicine or treatment. We got more familiar in Arizona with the medical, and the law that was coming down the pipe, and we wanted to be involved. So we applied to get our licence to grow in 2010 when our AMMA [*Arizona Medical Marijuana Act*] passed. We were awarded two grow licences, which allowed us the right to grow twelve plants each. Once we harvested over twenty pounds of flower, I realized I was going to have a real hard time smoking all that before the next harvest, so we turned it into food. That's where Zonka was born. We decided that we would start with a line of candy bars. Candy and chocolate are good carriers—easy to hide any bad aftertaste, and it's easy to implement for [*sick*] children, the elderly, and people with eating disorders. So we launched with six flavoured candy bars, which quickly grew to suckers, brownies, moon pies, Rice Krispie treats, cookies . . . Any way we could offer it, I tried it.

Journalist Ray Stern: Chris, being the pioneer that he is, developed this Zonka bar that patients wanted. They actually checked to see if people had medical marijuana cards or medical notes from the doctor because he was trying to do it right . . . Thousands of patients were buying at these compassion clubs, but no one was being busted for it because everyone kind of understood . . . that medical marijuana was here to stay. Now, in Yavapai County, they have taken this ridiculous extreme view against the voters . . . I spoke with Jack Fields, chief of the civil division at the time . . . and no surprise, he took the view that nothing like this could occur. And so, until the state issued actual dispensary licenses to people, no one was supposed to be selling marijuana and they were going to prosecute anyone that was.

Chris—September, 2012: The kids got up, we got dressed, we left for school, and not until I hit Highway 69 did I realize there was something completely weird about the morning. There were at least twelve marked and unmarked sheriff's officer cars, and they literally one by one followed suit as we went down the highway. Each mile we progressed down the highway, we had a longer parade behind us. The kids were catching on. They didn't know what was happening, but it was so deafening quiet in the car.

Andi: Me, I'm completely lost, because we have an attorney. I know we have this Zonka, but our attorney says it's fine. So that's not even crossing my mind. Not one time. That fifteen minutes felt like three hours.

Chris: Before I know it, an ambulance stopped all traffic and boom, my truck gets hit.

Andi: There were cops everywhere. And they're screaming, "Felony warrants! Felony warrants!" And Chris is gone, and I see the car is in drive, so I just went to put the car in park. [*An officer*] grabbed my hair and pulled me backwards. I looked back at the kids, and when we started the ride, they were each in their seatbelts, and there were three kids, but when I turned back and looked at them, it was like they were just one kid. They had all squished together. And a man in a suit had a huge assault rifle and went into the back seat where the kids were, and he grabbed my daughter's shoulder, and he full-bodied went in there and was screaming at them, "Give us your cell phones!" That's where I learned that I had really small arms and I came right out of the handcuffs. I remember kicking and screaming, "Those are KIDS!"

And all I want to know is where is Chris and what the hell is going on??

[*An associate working with Chris had replied to an email from an undercover police officer and sold over $1,000 in Zonka products without checking for a medicinal marijuana license. This was the conclusion of a $2 million investigation into Chris and the Desert Eagles Motorcycle Club. Law enforcement in their small town were members of a rival motorcycle club.*

Chris was charged with multiple felonies and was facing 127 years in prison for
- *Participation in a criminal syndicate*
- *2 counts marijuana violation*
- *Narcotic drug violation [for cannabis concentrates]*
- *Dangerous drug violation*
- *Drug paraphernalia violation*
- *4 counts misconduct weapons*
- *3 counts child endangerment*

With what Chris feels was true divine intervention, his bail was reduced from $250,000 to $50,000. In September of 2012, Chris was released on bond and Andi on her own recognizance. The Desert Eagles Motorcycle Club disbanded at the end of 2012. Chris and Andi decided to get into CBD because it was still medicinal, but legal, starting their edibles company, Hempful Farms CBD. Chris's goal was to build a business that would keep his family afloat when he went to prison.]

August 31, 2015—Chris's Sentencing: [*The plea was two years, and the sentence was handed down pretty quickly.*] My response was to ball it up and throw it on the floor. Like, you're crazy. I'm not admitting to anything when I never sold anything to a cop. I never did anything that I thought was illegal, according to the AMMA, so why would I admit it now?

But my lawyer took it as a sign that they were

retreating, when they gave us the two-year plea. My lawyer pulled me outside and said, "Wait, wait. Before you deny this plea, realize that they are handing you the white flag. They're throwing in the towel. They're stating that you won."

Strike me as a weirdo, but it's hard to feel like a winner when I'm admitting guilt, and I'm going to prison, leaving my family. But when he says, "The alternative is we go to trial, and we fight for you just like you want me to, and the same fourteen that indicted you find you guilty, and then you go for thirty, and you call my office every day crying because you want to go home, and I don't take the call, and then you're really mad at me, because that's real life. So, if that's the option, and that's what you'd like to do, because that's how this system works, then go for it."

My first nickname in prison was Hollywood. And I got that name because of how much mail I received. It was just one more awesome thing that my wife did. My wife really was the key support system.

Andi: When Chris left for prison, I ended up taking over Hempful Farms. I moved the business to my house; I had to make all the products at home. I couldn't afford staff anymore, so it was me and the kids. We would rent a kitchen so that we could still be in compliance, using a commercial kitchen. I did all the shipping, ran all the marketing. It wasn't just my job—one, I love doing what I do, and two, I love my family. And so because we believe so strongly in what we do, you can do anything. I didn't think I could. I thought that when Chris left, that was it. I thought I wasn't going to be able to keep it going. He was the one who knew how to market. He was the face, and I was behind the scenes, so I really thought I was going to lose it. But I did it. And I had Chris. Every day, our fifteen minutes, it might have been ten minutes of work talk. And in our letters, he would remind me

of what the hashtags were, when I needed to make a post. So he helped me. [*Andi smiles.*]

Chris: You know, there were two valuable lessons taught to us from this. My wife is very passive, in the background. And me, I've gotta control and run everything. You go to prison and you lose all that ability. So the two lessons we learned were I need to shut up. Slow down. Realize what I've got Andi for. And Andi realized how important she is to this business and this family. We can't do this without her. This chick did everything, from pitches, to *The Marijuana Show*, to running the company from $3,000 a month in sales to $100,000 a month. By herself. With a *six year old*. I mean. What *didn't* she do? I think that's probably an easier question to answer.

The funniest part—how do you love somebody more today than then? My mom didn't show me that—my dad, my family, the marriages didn't show me that. But my best friend showed me that. And I will never be able to repay that.

February 21, 2017—Chris is released from prison: All I know is walking out of that prison and seeing a family that was tortured. And knowing that each step was one step away, and one step forward, to THIS. And to the future. I don't think I'll ever be able to relive that. I don't think I'll ever be able to touch on those emotions, and those feelings. But I can tell you that a fire was lit in there. And it will not burn out.

At the end of the day, all the bullshit aside, and the negativity, and the crookedness, and all the evil that people focus on. At the end of the day, it's really about the changes that are being made. Just because of this—because of this movement. So just don't give up. Don't quit. Ever. I've been at that ledge, on one toe. And never thought I'd be here.

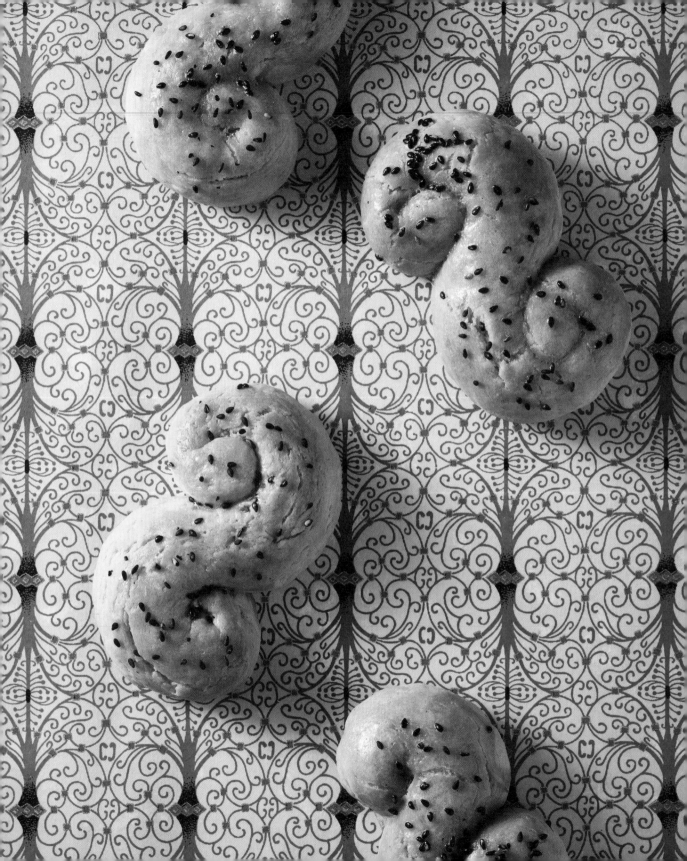

Greek Koulourakia

Easier than spelling Koulourakia, this special recipe emerged from my
brother-in-law's sister's childhood notebook; Lena had written the recipe in
pencil after having made it with her Greek grandmother. Lena is all grown
up now and open to people's use of cannabis, especially if it may relieve
anxiety or assist with relief from substance use disorders.
Lena is an RN at a supervised injection site.

SUGGESTED MOOD/STRAIN

Greek Kalamata is a hard-hitting
sativa known for encouraging
focus. Although it's not known to
be a prominent pain reliever, it is
said to help with migraines.

Makes 30 koulourakia with ½ cup
cannabutter (almost 5 mg THC
per cookie).

½ cup (113 g) cannabutter
½ cup (113 g) unsalted butter,
   room temperature
1 cup (200 g) granulated sugar
6 egg yolks + 1 additional egg
   reserved for egg wash
2½ tsp baking soda
2½ tsp baking powder
1 lemon, zested and juiced
2 tsp vanilla extract
¼ cup (63 mL) milk
About 4 cups (568 g) all-purpose
   flour + additional for working
   with the dough
2–3 Tbsp roasted black sesame
   seeds

Preheat the oven to 350°F and prepare baking sheet(s) with
parchment paper or silicone mat(s).

Melt the cannabutter in a double boiler or in a heat-proof
bowl over a pot of simmering water.

With your favourite mixer, combine the butters and sugar.
Add the yolks, one at a time, scraping down the bowl regularly.

In another bowl, add the baking soda and baking powder to
the lemon juice (it will fizz), and pour into the butter and sugar
mixture. Add the zest, vanilla, and milk.

Add the flour a little at a time. If the dough is too soft to work
with, add a little more. (When ready, it will still be a sticky dough,
but you'll be able to mould it.)

Mark off 8 inches on a flat surface. Grab a lump of dough
that's about 1½ Tbsp, and roll it out into a thick 8-inch worm.
You can form whatever shapes you might like for your cookies,
but there are a few traditional shapes. One is a swirly "S" shape,
where the ends curl in on themselves in opposite directions.
Another is a closed tuning-fork shape, flipped into a few twists.
The "S" shape is easier to achieve without breakage because you
don't have to lift the dough. Whatever shape(s) you choose,
continue to work the rest of the dough into cookies, placing the
results onto the baking sheets. (They will puff up a little, so space
them a healthy inch or two apart.)

Brush the cookies with egg using a pastry brush or new paint
brush, and sprinkle with the sesame seeds.

Bake for 15–20 minutes until gently browned.

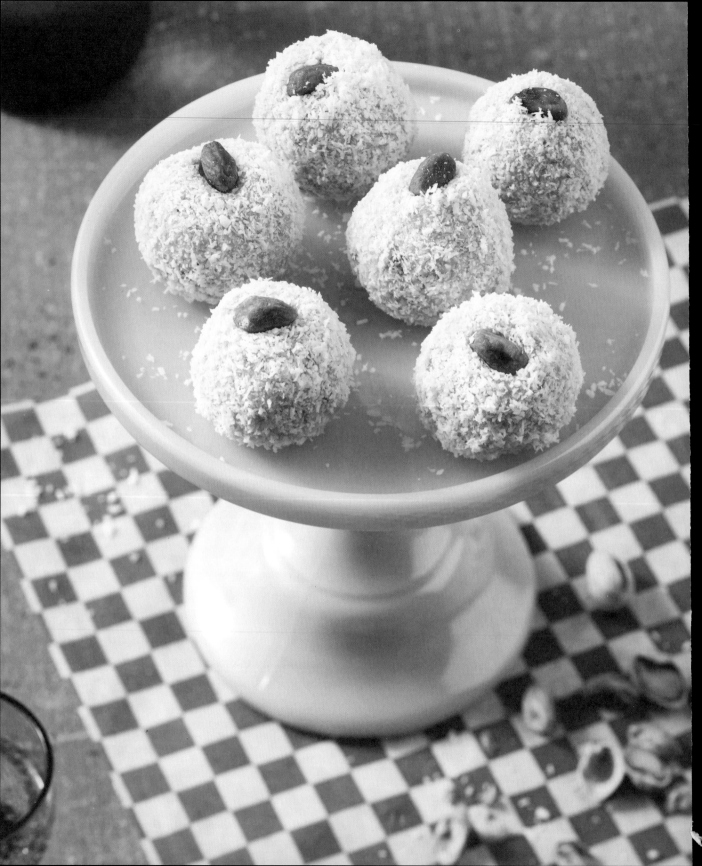

Coconut Laddoos

Much easier than desiccating a coconut, this recipe is based on an IG post by Rinku Sharma, @bongcookingstory. Rinku's gorgeous little white coco treats for Janmashtami, the Hindu festival celebrating the birth of Lord Krishna, immediately caught my attention. Janmashtami is celebrated on the eighth day of the month Bhadrapada (August or September), and prayers are offered to Lord Krishna with offerings of sweets. I encourage you to follow Rinku on IG.

SUGGESTED MOOD/STRAIN

Andhra Bhang comes from the Bay of Bengal in India, giving a "cerebral" high.

Makes 16 laddoos with ¼ cup cannaghee (almost 5 mg THC per piece).

¼ cup (57 g) cannaghee*

3 cups (270 g) finely shredded unsweetened coconut, divided

1 can (300 mL) sweetened condensed milk

½ cup (63 g) pistachios, chopped in a food processor or by hand (some large bits reserved)

Melt the cannaghee in a frying pan.

Stir in 2 cups of coconut. Fry for a bit over low heat, trying not to brown, stirring constantly for 2 or 3 minutes.

Add in the sweetened condensed milk. Stir with a wooden spoon for about 5 minutes until the "dough" comes together. Don't let the mixture dry out.

Stir in the pistachios, reserving some bigger pieces for garnishing.

When the dough has cooled enough to handle but is still warm, roll and squeeze it into golf ball–sized balls.

Roll and shower each ball in the reserved 1 cup of coconut and press a reserved pistachio piece into the top of each ball.

*Ghee is clarified butter. It works better than traditional butter in this recipe because the milk solids would otherwise brown, causing the laddoos to lose their snowy-white colour. (Ask me how I know.) You can make your own ghee (Google it) or purchase it, and then make cannaghee from it following the same directions as for cannabutter (page 26). Some say that removing the milk solids also increases the potency of cannabutter.

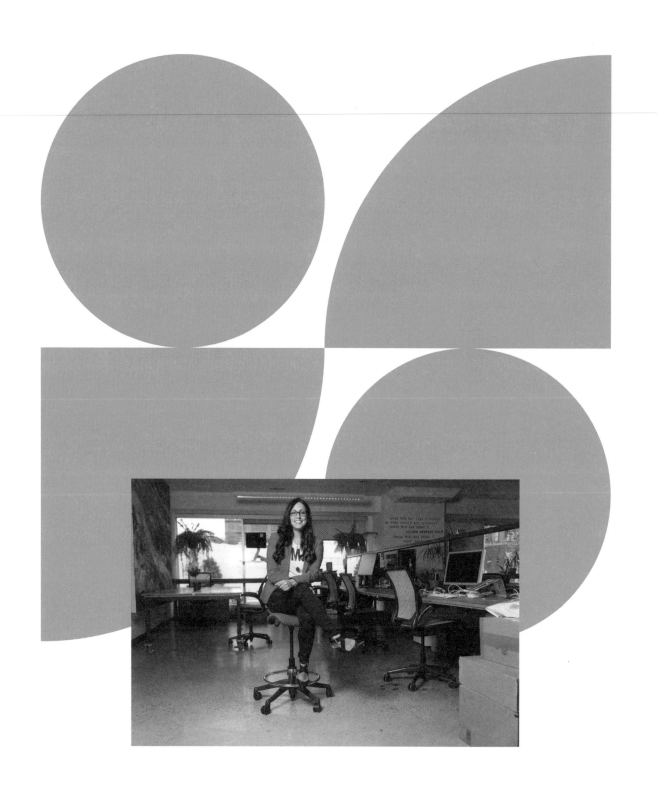

Cynthia Salarizadeh

Cynthia Salarizadeh is founder and president of the luxury infused beverages company House of Saka, founder of the technology platform MediaSphere, and co-founder of Green Market Media, a cannabis industry-focused public relations and consulting firm based in California. She is also the entrepreneur behind the tech suite AxisWire, as well as the co-founder of the women's cannabis leadership network Industry Power Women.

Okay, so I smoked weed, I think, starting at the end of my senior year of high school for the first time. I've always been pretty open to it, but, you know, I was raised in New Jersey, so for us, it was always something very illegal. The possibility of it ever even being something we could have walked into a store and bought was never even a thought for us. But, time passed, and I decided that I wanted to finish my college degree because I kept hitting every ceiling professionally without it, so I went to community college to clean up my GPA in order to apply for the University of Pennsylvania, and the very first paper that I wrote, almost five years before Colorado even thought about recreational cannabis, was a fifteen-page paper on legalizing cannabis. I wrote about what it would do for our economy and what it would do for the medical community. And then I didn't think about that paper again until after entering the industry.

I should mention that around that same time, my brother was suffering from an opiate addiction. It started out with Percocet, and evolved into Oxycontin. And when you can't afford a one thousand dollar a day habit, that turns into heroin. And unfortunately, like many people caught in that epidemic, my brother passed away. Our family was, understandably, gutted. When you go through something traumatic like that, it really does change absolutely everything about your perspective on life and how we manage what we put into our bodies.

Not too long afterward, I transferred to the University of Pennsylvania. I wrote my senior thesis on Big Oil and sustainable economic development, and in its conclusion, I realized that one of the only possibilities for us to reduce our dependency on fossil fuels was through industrial hemp. When I graduated, I thought I'd go straight into the State Department, but instead, I immediately got an offer from my friends who had started a technology start-up called CannaFundr. I was at a real crossroads. At first, my friends' offer seemed silly, professionally. It was a huge risk to enter the cannabis field. I was told I'd never be able to go back to corporate America, that I would never be able to work with the DOD [*Department of Defense*] or the State Department. That's literally what I was told.

But then my father sat me down and said that I had a skill set that could advance this particular industry, and just to take a couple of years to give it a shot. That was weird, because my dad has never smoked a cigarette and he's against drugs. He was a master chief in the Navy. So I figured there had to be a reason why he was telling me this. I assumed maybe he was trying to dissuade me from the other paths I was considering; I simply didn't know. So I spent a couple months researching everything. Personally, it felt like accepting my friends' offer was the right thing to do. Because if I could just help for a couple years, then other families wouldn't have to go through what our family had gone through, and then I'd have done my part. So I did. I entered the industry. For me, the decision was personal. If it had been professional, I never would have done it.

[I asked Cynthia if she could help explain the connection between losing her brother to opioids and feeling that entering the cannabis industry might help other families.]

Well, the only drug that the world can figure out to help reduce dependency on opiates, to properly try for withdrawal, is cannabis. It might have provided an opportunity or a chance for my brother that he simply didn't have in another way. There's another drug out there called kratom that's also natural and might be able to help opiate addicts. But of course, the government has made it illegal. So between the cannabis and the kratom, there is a chance my brother would have at least had a path to truly try to kick the addiction.

About two months ago, a study was released saying that in states where there is recreational or medical marijuana—where there are marijuana programs—opiate addiction has gone down 30 percent. So I can sleep better at night, knowing the path that I selected helped make this happen. That was my goal, and between all of the people set out to do just this . . . it worked. I joined the industry, and in the end, it wound up being the best possible decision I ever could have made. I can never thank my father enough for convincing me. Here I thought I was being rejected from something, but somehow my dad knew that this was going to be big and amazing, and now I sit at the centre of it.

Because of the area I had worked in, public relations, I had my hands in everything. I worked with every type of company, every type of person who was involved in the industry, and I got a front-row seat to where all the trends were going. Before the pandemic, I produced the *Cannabis Trend Report* every year. And when I'd create those reports, I'd notice there were wide open lanes and opportunities, and if I had the resources to make something happen without taking on investment, I'd try it. I launched the news site because that was fairly easy to do without investment. I launched the newswire, which was also a major need for the industry at that time, and in fact, when we started to build the technology, the newswires that existed in regular industries wouldn't even allow us to publish the terms "marijuana" or "cannabis." Now, I'm getting ready to launch my final company in cannabis, a communications platform we've been building for three years.

The only company that actually took investment to even launch was the [*alcohol-free*] cannabis wine, the luxury brand House of Saka. The term "Saka" is interchangeable with the "Scythians," the Central Asian tribe of a couple thousand years ago, where the mythological Amazonians, the Wonder Women, came from. It was an Iranian tribe, and I'm Persian, so the name of the brand is special to me. And we're an all-female crew. Collectively, we have hundreds of years of wine experience, a ridiculous amount of cannabis experience, and more importantly, the beverages just taste amazing.

And on that note, there's a ton of opportunity in cannabis for women. Where in other industries it's already saturated and you're fighting against titans, in cannabis, we do have titans now, but there are maybe only four or five big ones still to this day. If anything, that benefits you in the industry because the titans can come and acquire you if you need them.

But there are definitely problems. Taxation and banking are the two biggest challenges for any cannabis business, entrepreneur, operator, or whatever the case may be. The SAFE Banking Act just made it through another step, and we actually think it might go through sometime soon, but as of now, we're not allowed to use banks here, in the United States. It's all cash, and we have to deliver the cash to the banks, and deliver our taxation in cash. It's bizarre, and more importantly, dangerous. And I don't know if you've ever spoken to anybody who has put in an application for a licence? But it's equal to the stress of writing a one-hundred-page thesis. I can't even begin to describe the challenges, just in that part. If you think the underground growers are going to sit and do that, you're crazy.

And with beverages, at this time, two years into the new beverage infusion technology, which allows for the cannabis beverages we now see everywhere,

California still only has one manufacturer for every beverage brand. *One.* And it's killing us. You go to Michigan, and there are thirty large manufacturing facilities with state-of-the-art equipment. It's just shocking what's going on in other states, while California is just stumbling along. Of course, we've got the best growers outside of Colombia and maybe Uruguay, but other than cultivation in the Emerald Triangle, we're still struggling. The laws are still a mess, manufacturing is a mess, distribution is the biggest mess ever, and sampling is horrible. I have to paint our bottles because there's a law that you can't have clear beverage containers (that was a steep cost per bottle!), and we've had to put this ugly black child-proof cap on top. One day we woke up and were told we couldn't put "Napa Valley" on our bottles anymore. Do you know how much money we spend to use Napa Valley wine? Now we can't even label it that. Every day it's something different. It's just one hurdle after the next with cannabis. It never ends.

But at the same time, I would never wish for anything different. I have no idea if I ever would have become some form of serial entrepreneur if I had been in a different industry. I would have just stuck with my PR firm and that would have been it.

But in this industry, at this time, there was just so much opportunity. If I hadn't taken a chance, what kind of person would I be?

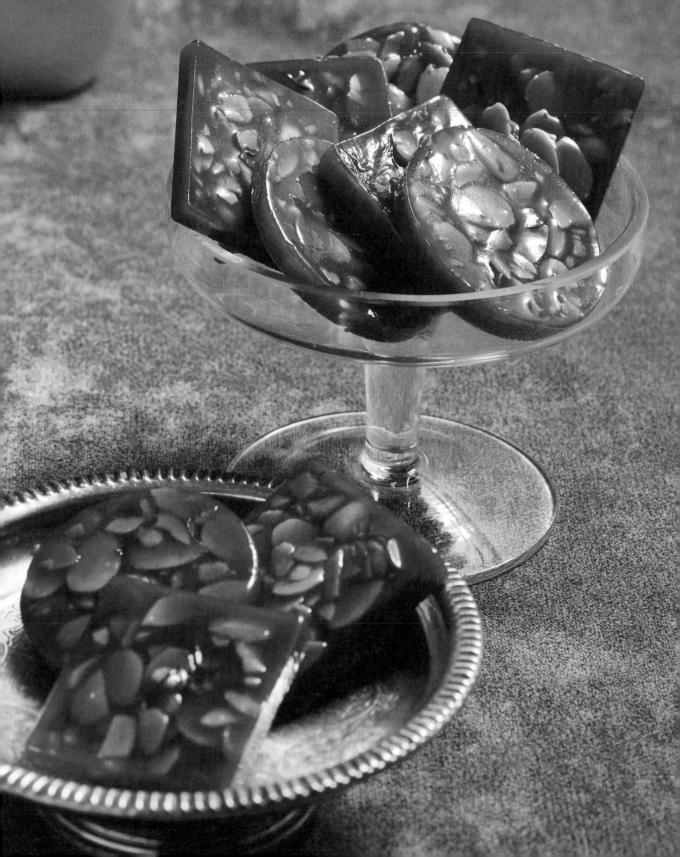

Persian-Style Honey Saffron Brittle

This recipe is easier than figuring out if you've been scammed by fake saffron. Hint—the real stuff doesn't come in a big batch, and it's really expensive! Only 3 little fibres come from each flower and they're harvested by hand. It takes 1,000 flowers to get 1 ounce of saffron.

SUGGESTED MOOD/STRAIN

Iranian is a landrace from Khorasan, a historic region partially in modern Iran with high bud production. The Muslim mystic who is believed to have discovered hash was from Khorasan.

Makes 13 candies with 3 Tbsp cannabutter (about 4 mg THC per piece).

1 cup (200 g) granulated sugar
2 Tbsp honey
3 Tbsp (43 g) cannabutter
1 Tbsp rosewater*
½ cup (63 g) sliced almonds
1 tsp saffron**
Half a lemon, juiced
2 or 3 drops of red food colouring
Cooking spray

Be sure to measure all ingredients ahead so that you can just throw things in as needed once you get your candy factory going.

Whisk the sugar, honey, and cannabutter together on the stove over low heat until the sugar melts, about 5 or 10 minutes.

Add the rosewater and continue to stir until the mix goes slightly golden brown, another minute or so. Clip on that candy thermometer.

Stir in the almonds. The mix should begin to thicken a little. Let it go until you get to the "hard crack" (300° to 310°F) stage on the candy thermometer.

Finally, add in the saffron, lemon juice, and food colouring. Let this cook about a minute, making sure the temp is back to hard crack, and then use a ladle or large spoon to divide syrup into the compartments of a silicone cupcake tray sprayed liberally with cooking spray. Soak your tools and saucepan right away to avoid a super glue situation.

Chill for about an hour if you can stand to wait, and then enjoy your candy.

*Rosewater can be found at your favourite diverse grocery store or online.

**You're probably saying, "Ann, I have to hunt for two specialty ingredients in one recipe?" Pipe down—do you want to transport your tongue to the Middle East or not? I found some cheaper-than-usual saffron at everyone's favourite suburban box store! (Wink.)

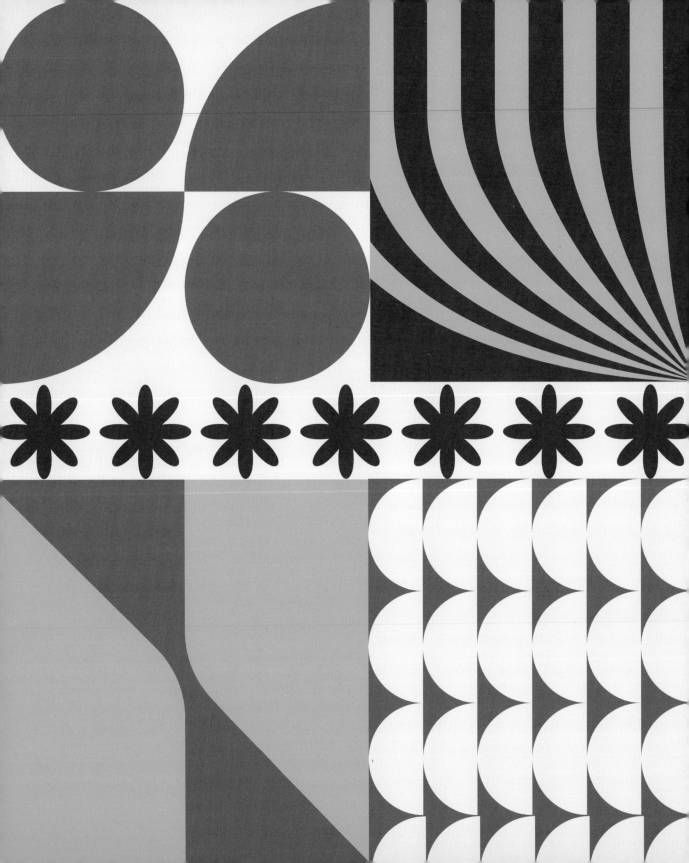

NUTTY

RECIPES

STORIES

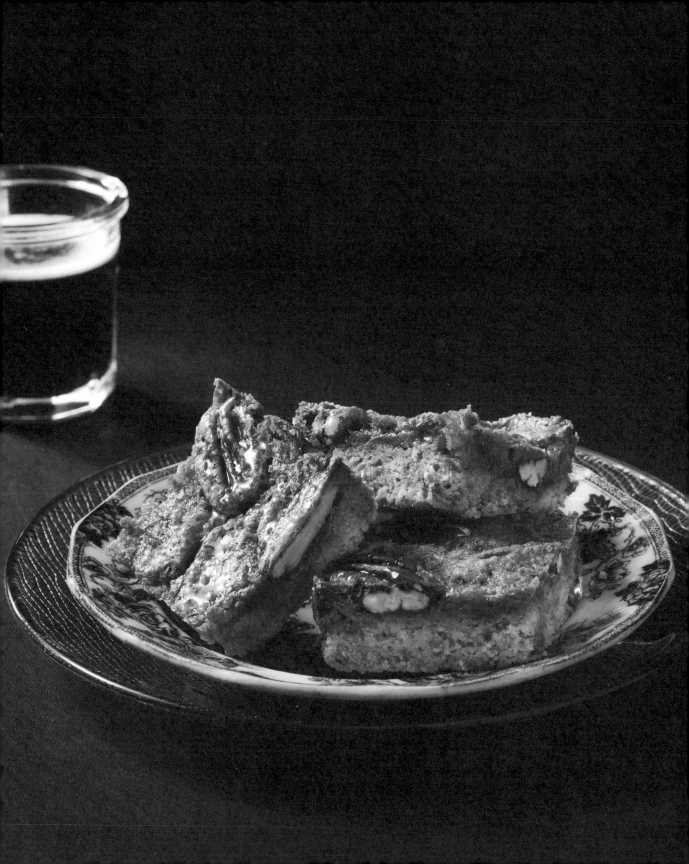

Pecan Pie Squares

Easier than pronouncing it pe-cahn while insisting you're still Jenny from the Block.

SUGGESTED MOOD/STRAIN

Pecan Bubba is just the cutest name for a cannabis strain ever. I know nothing else about it.

Makes 12 squares with ¼ cup cannabutter (about 6 mg THC per piece).

Crust
¼ cup (57 g) cannabutter
¼ cup (57 g) unsalted butter, room temperature
¼ cup (50 g) superfine granulated sugar
1⅔ cups (237 g) all-purpose flour
Dash of salt
Cooking spray

Filling
½ cup (125 mL) corn syrup
½ cup (125 mL) honey
1½ cups (300 g) brown sugar
2 eggs
½ cup (113 g) butter, melted
2 tsp vanilla extract
2 Tbsp whipping (35%) cream
¼ cup (36 g) all-purpose flour

Topping
1½ cups (190 g) pretty pecans

Preheat oven to 350°F.

Melt the cannabutter in a double boiler or in a heat-proof bowl over a pot of simmering water. With your favourite mixer, combine the crust ingredients. Press to uniform thickness in the sections of a squares pan prepped with cooking spray, or in the bottom of an 8 × 8–inch pan lined with parchment paper that also extends up 2 sides for "handles."* Bake for about 8 minutes until the crust gently browns.

While the crust is baking, whisk together the filling ingredients. Spoon the filling on top of the crust(s) and top with pecans.

Bake for 20–25 minutes until bubbly. Allow the squares to cool completely (in the fridge) before removing from the pan, loosening all edges carefully with a knife; this will be a b&tch if they stick, but go ahead and smack it upside-down on the counter. Slice with a sharp knife if you used a square pan.

*A squares pan (looks like a muffin pan but with 12 squares) will give a cleaner result for this recipe. If you insist, though, an 8 × 8 or 9 × 9–inch square pan will totally work instead. If using a 9 × 9, increase ingredients by 25 percent.

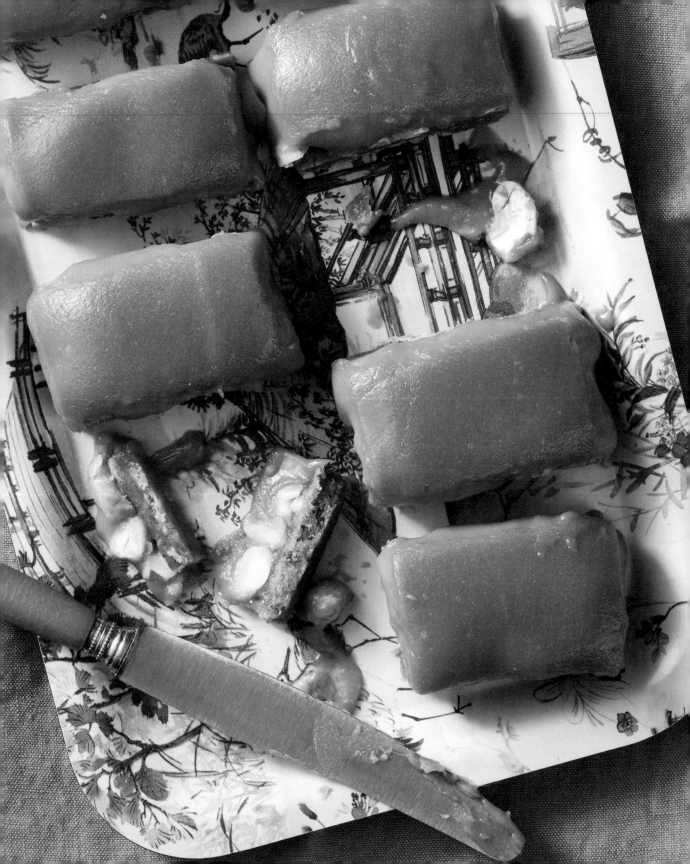

Butterscotch Cashew Pudding Squares

This recipe is easier than explaining the difference between caramel and butterscotch (which is actually very easy—caramel is made with white sugar while butterscotch is made with brown).

Makes 16 squares with ¼ cup cannabutter (almost 5 mg THC per piece).

Crust

Oil
¼ cup (57 g) cannabutter
¼ cup (57 g) unsalted butter, room
   temperature
½ cup (100 g) brown sugar
1 cup (142 g) all-purpose flour
Dash of salt

Filling

6 Tbsp (85 g) unsalted butter
6 Tbsp (53 g) all-purpose flour
1 cup (200 g) brown sugar
2 cups (500 mL) milk
2 tsp vanilla extract
3 egg yolks
1 cup (127 g) cashews, chopped

Preheat oven to 350°F and prepare an 8 × 8–inch baking pan with oil or butter, lining the bottom with parchment paper overhanging on two sides (to be used as handles).

Melt the cannabutter in a double boiler or in a heat-proof bowl over a pot of simmering water.

With your favourite mixer, combine all crust ingredients, starting with the butters and sugar and ending with the flour and salt. Press the cookie dough crust evenly into the pan.

Bake for about 12 minutes until the crust dries up a little and turns light brown.

While the crust is cooking, get the filling going. In a medium heavy-bottomed pot, melt the butter, and add the flour. Stir around over medium-low heat for a minute or two.

Add the brown sugar and milk. Bring to a boil, whisking fairly constantly, then turn the heat to medium-low again and whisk regularly while the filling cooks for the next 10 minutes. Add the vanilla in the final minute or so.

Remove the filling from the heat and, very ferociously, whisk in the egg yolks. Cook while whisking for a few minutes more.

Sprinkle the crust with the chopped cashews and pour the filling overtop evenly. Let the pan cool on the counter until just warm, when you can transfer it to the fridge to chill completely.

Loosen the goodness from the edges of the pan with a thin knife. Use the parchment handles to lift the butterscotch slab to a flat surface, then peel the parchment off. Use a heavy knife to cut into quarters and quarters again, ending up with 16 squares. These will be a little messy; serve in small dishes with forks.

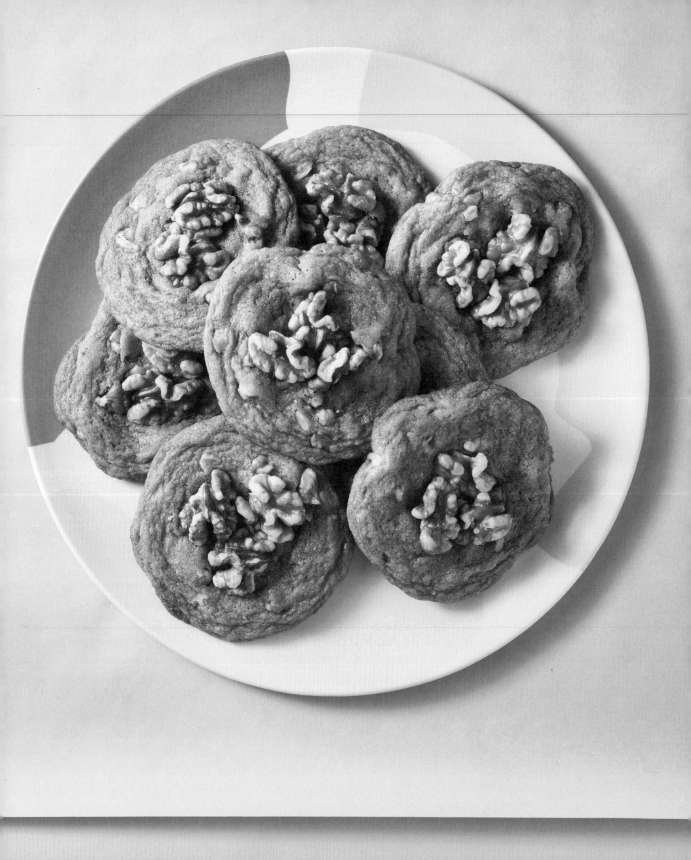

Maple Walnut Cookies

Easier than tapping a maple tree. Like, much easier.

Maple Leaf Indica "is a heroic strain of Indica with fat leaves, plump buds, and caked with crystals," according to *Leafly*. Sounds delicious!

Makes about 28 cookies with ½ cup cannabutter (about 5 mg THC per piece).

½ cup (113 g) cannabutter
1 cup (200 g) brown sugar
1 egg
½ cup (125 mL) real maple syrup
1 tsp maple extract
1¾ cups (249 g) all-purpose flour
1 tsp baking powder
½ tsp baking soda
Dash of salt
1¾ cups (222 g) walnuts (¾ cups chopped; 1 cup walnut halves, tossed in olive oil and salt)

Preheat oven to 375°F and line baking sheet(s) with parchment paper or silicone mat(s).

Melt the cannabutter in a double boiler or in a heat-proof bowl over a pot of simmering water.

With your favourite mixer, combine the cannabutter and brown sugar. Add in the egg. Next go for the maple syrup and extract.

In a separate bowl, stir together the flour, baking powder, baking soda, and salt. Add the dry ingredients to the mixing bowl. Add the ¾ cup chopped walnuts.

With a 1-Tbsp cookie scoop, drop dough onto the baking sheet(s). These cookies will spread, so make sure they're at least 1½ inches apart. Bake for 6–8 minutes.

While the cookies are baking, toast the remaining walnuts in the microwave. In a microwave-safe bowl, nuke the pretty walnut halves in 2-minute increments until they start to smell lovely (no more than 6 minutes).

The cookies are done when there isn't a mound of dough in the middle, but they're not completely cooked either. Bang the cookies two or three times on the counter to flatten them. If they don't flatten, give them another 2 minutes in the oven. Decorate the cookie centres with 3 pretty toasted walnut halves on each cookie while they're still warm.

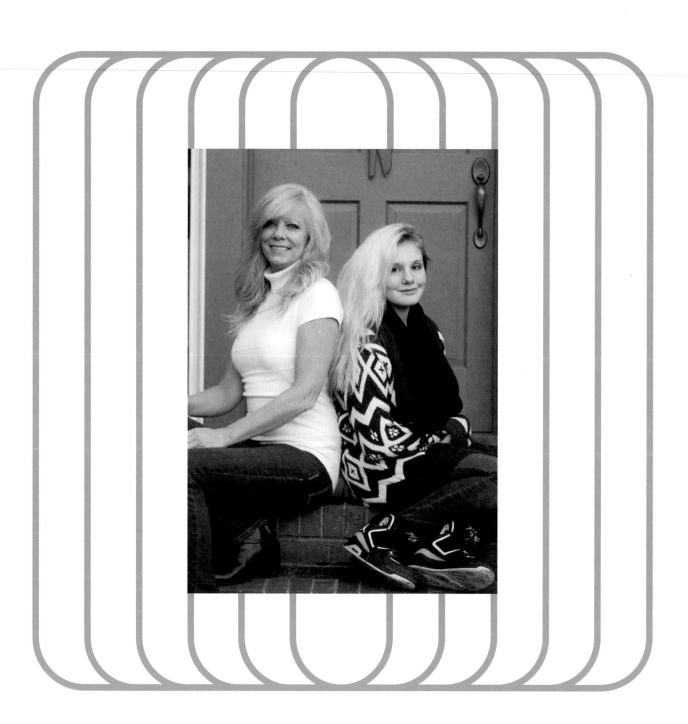

Al Bryant

Al Bryant became a cannabis activist after having to acquire it illegally for her mother, who died of colon cancer five years ago. Al and her mother were living in North Carolina, where, at time of writing, possession of 14 to 42 grams (½ to 1½ ounces) of cannabis is a misdemeanor and greater than 42 grams is a felony. Cultivation of any amount of cannabis is a Class 1 felony. There are no exceptions in the state's law for medicinal use. Al herself is a survivor and medicinal user; her cancer is currently in remission.

I was sixteen years old when we found out. My mother had been putting off going to the doctor for a few years prior to her diagnosis; we were in Wilmington, North Carolina, when we found out that she had Stage 2 stomach cancer. And then after having two surgeries in Wilmington, and two in Winston-Salem, she was about to go into remission from the stomach cancer but found out that the cancer had spread to her colon, "promoting" her to Stage 3. Soon enough, because she was given the wrong chemo and too little of it, the cancer progressed to Stage 4. She was a lawyer and had been accepted to the North Carolina General Assembly two months prior to when she died, but she was too sick to do anything about that. In the end, she moved again to Marion, North Carolina, to be closer to my grandparents, and she passed away there after about three weeks, almost four.

And, honestly, I don't even mind saying this anymore, because, you know, I was seventeen at the time, but . . . I would have to help her buy weed. I knew people from high school and then . . . you know . . . that age group, when you're already doing that kind of stuff . . . And there was no access to any medicine. My mom was too sick to take the painkillers at that point because they just make you throw up. And if you throw up with a colostomy bag, you are literally throwing up feces, and spreading more infection throughout your body. So you know, that's not good. All those medicines related to the radiation and chemo, they make you so sick. And nobody truly understands that until you go through it.

But after a bit of weed, the nausea would stop. You know, it was hard to watch, because most of the time my mom would be in bed, curled up in a ball, because she just couldn't move. And then when she had the weed, that was the only time I'd see her sit up. And she would be smiling. She wouldn't say much; she was in much pain. But she wouldn't be whimpering. She wouldn't be holding back winces, little cries of agony. That would almost instantly stop, after the first two, three hits. And then she'd be able to lay back down and rest peacefully without, you know, being bent over a bucket, trying not to throw up, which is all she would do for months. That medicine truly, I believe, had a huge impact on her. And I can stand firm that it has definitely also saved my life, or has at least made a huge improvement. At five years old, I had fibrosarcoma and lost my right collarbone to it, and unfortunately, fibrosarcoma always comes back. It's not a chance of "if"—it's just a matter of when. It usually returns within five or ten years. And with how much I do smoke a day [*Al laughs*], I believe that's what has kept the tumour at bay for this long.

[*So cannabis isn't legal at all in North Carolina? Even medicinally?*]

Nope. Not at all.

Like I said, I was able to help my mom with medicine when we were near home, because I knew people in high school. But later, it was harder for me to get it for her, because I only knew Wilmington and Chapel Hill people. So at the end of her life, when she went to Marion, I knew nobody. And she knew nobody. So that was just tragic to deal with. I don't believe that anybody should have to deal with that. They should be allowed to go through dispensaries, and absolutely be given . . . not even just cancer patients, medically, but a number of other qualifying patients, like with glaucoma, or HIV, cystic fibrosis. Any one of those, and more, should have access.

Right now we're fighting for it, and there are a few bills up in the Senate. The one that's doing the best is HB711, which is an absolute joke. It's the "Compassionate Care Act," and it covers about eight things, and they've taken off four major qualifications that would really benefit people, one of them being glaucoma. And there are four dispensaries—it was cut from eight to four—that will need a $10K licence, and then the start-up cost to even open a business, that's like, another $50K, so I think that is absolutely criminal, that that's even brought to the table. But it's the only [*bill*] that's reaching the furthest, because government has the most control over it, is what I think.

Throughout North Carolina, it's not about the people, it's more about control. And I don't think personally it will ever get better. The state failed my mom, and even me, being a survivor. In any other state, when you say that you are a cancer survivor, they literally speed up your paperwork through the system so that you get your card sooner. Half the time the doctor will write you a prescription on a piece of paper that says that while your card is coming in the mail, there's a written prescription and your allotted medicinal cannabis, enabling you to the discounts and the higher quantities, and you're able to grow more at home, so that you can have it available. But cutting those people out of the picture, I just think that's sad, while they're being fed prescription pad after prescription pad of opiates. They're just left there to drool on themselves, wondering if this is the rest of their life now.

Also, veterans. That's a big one. North Carolina has the top suicide rate, almost out of any state in the U.S., for veteran suicide related to opiates or other prescription painkillers, and we also have some of the highest incarceration rates for cannabis. Even though cannabis is decriminalized on a very low scale, which is a joke, it's half an ounce or under. But even then, the fine is about two hundred to five hundred dollars, and that still gets you community service, or some type of probation. I just don't understand that. Even Texas has a medicinal bill. Idaho is considering it. Even Ohio, the state that everyone hates the most, probably, has a medicinal bill that is very inclusive, with generalized anxiety and depression, which I think is very important. Yes, SSRIs do help, but nobody wants to walk around in a zombie-like coma from Xanax. I mean, I don't, personally. Luckily, we do have CBD, though? But you know, sorry, it's mids. It's good for anxiety and depression, but it's just not pain relieving. People argue for it, and fight for it, and

I understand where they're coming from, and I guess if you smoke or eat enough of it then you'll get some kind of effect similar to ibuprofen, maybe, but I still think that's an absolute joke. It's very, very limited in this state, and it has been for years.

Financially, for my mother, things were also terrible. The house went into foreclosure because we weren't able to pay it off. I had to leave Wilmington. There was barely any inheritance. I did recover some funds through our malpractice settlement, but I can never recover my mom's life, or our home in Wilmington.

This was also when North Carolina was going through the HB2 "Bathroom" Bill. All the music, TV shows, and movies they were making here got cut, because transgenders were restricted from using their preferred bathroom or the one related to their identity. That really made a lot of people angry, including me. But because of that bill, every act that was coming to North Carolina cancelled. Most importantly, for me, was Bruce Springsteen, because I was supposed to see him with my mom, one more time, before she passed away. [*Al struggles to get this out through tears.*] I saw him twice in concert with her when his saxophone player was still alive. But the tickets were refunded, and I don't even know if he's been back to North Carolina since. He used to love coming to Raleigh, Durham, Charlotte. And that bill had a huge effect on the state; it went pretty much almost broke, because lawyers in North Carolina get paid by the state. It doesn't matter if you work for yourself, if you work for a firm, you get paid mainly by the state. So when the state went broke, that really, really took a toll on my mom. In my opinion, we should never have left Illinois. Ever. I have a lot of hostility toward North Carolina. And that's why I'm back [*from Illinois, where Al moved a few years after her mom passed*]. We have unfinished business.

[*What can people do to help fight, Al? In North Carolina, or if something similar is going on for them where they live?*]

Volunteering with NORML [*National Organization for the Reform of Marijuana Laws*] is a great idea. If there's any meeting, or orientation in your area, I'd say sign up for it, or follow their Instagram, Facebook, Twitter, or even their website. And then focus on your legislator—like, NC.gov, or whatever state you're in—to see what bills are being processed through. Keeping up-to-date on that, or even emailing your representatives, can get you further in getting your voice heard. A lot of times people think that their letters just go to the junk mail, but legally, they at least have to scan over them. They're required to see them.

I think change is coming. There was a federal bill presented not too long ago. I think it was about two weeks ago. And I'm trying to be realistic about it, but the fact that it's on the floor stands for something. Even if it doesn't go far, at least it got to the floor.

I'm back in North Carolina now, to try to fight for access to this medicine, for people like me and my mother. I've reached out to a few legislators and I've already gotten a positive response.

I'm hopeful, at least, that my mom knowing that her daughter is back fighting for her will make some kind of stance. I'm doing that because of who my mom was. That's what I'm really hoping for.

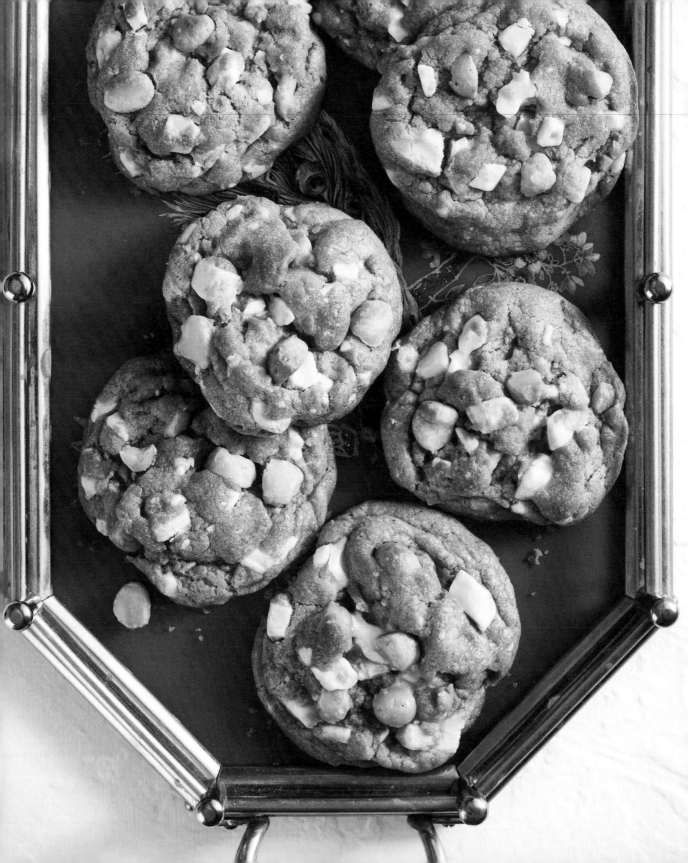

White Chocolate Macadamias with Amaretto

This recipe is easier than figuring out how the great macadamia made it from Australia to Hawaii and South Africa.

SUGGESTED MOOD/STRAIN

Amaretto Sour is a sativa-dominant hybrid that will leave you feeling energetic and rejuvenated.

Makes about 28 cookies with ½ cup cannabutter (about 5 mg THC per piece).

½ cup (113 g) cannabutter
½ cup (113 g) unsalted butter, melted
1½ cups (250 g) brown sugar
1 egg + 1 yolk
2¾ cups (284 g) all-purpose flour
1 tsp baking soda
Dash of salt
4 Tbsp amaretto
1 cup (160 g) white chocolate, chopped
½ cup (64 g) macadamia nuts

Preheat the oven to 350°F and prepare baking sheet(s) with parchment paper or silicone mat(s).

Melt the cannabutter in a double boiler or in a heat-proof bowl over a pot of simmering water.

With your favourite mixer, combine butters and brown sugar. Add in egg and yolk.

In a separate bowl, stir the flour, baking soda, and salt together. Add to the mixing bowl in a few additions. Add the amaretto.

If your mixer can handle it, add in the white chocolate and macadamias. If your mixer can't handle it, do this with a wooden spoon.

Using a 1-Tbsp cookie scoop, drop generous lumps of dough onto the baking sheet(s). Bake for about 10 minutes until the cookies lose their shine.

Remove cookies to a cooling rack and allow them to cool completely.

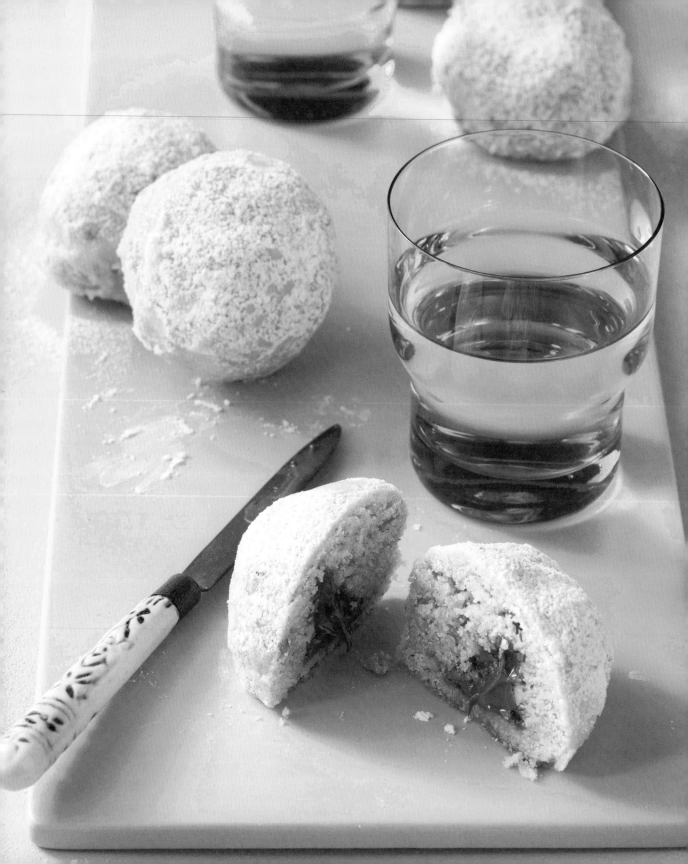

Snowballs

As easy as a snow job (if you don't know what that is, ask a Canadian).

SUGGESTED MOOD/STRAIN

Let's go with *Snow Bud*, an Afghan–South African hybrid.

Makes about 18 cookies with ¼ cup + 2 Tbsp cannabutter (about 6 mg THC per cookie).

18 tsp chocolatey hazelnut spread (sometimes of Italian origin, wink, wink)
¼ cup + 2 Tbsp (85 g) cannabutter
2 Tbsp (29 g) unsalted butter
1 cup (200 g) granulated sugar
1⅔ cups (160 g) almond flour
⅔ cups (85 g) pecans, chopped
1 tsp vanilla extract
1 tsp cayenne pepper
Icing (powdered) sugar, for coating

Dollop 18 1-tsp lumps of "chocolatey hazelnut spread" (wink) onto a baking sheet lined with parchment paper and freeze until solid, for at least 15 minutes.

Melt the cannabutter in a double boiler or in a heat-proof bowl over a pot of simmering water.

In a large bowl using a wooden spoon, combine the cannabutter and the rest of the ingredients, except for the icing sugar.

Remove the hazelnut bumps from the freezer and surround each with dough, forming golf-ball-sized balls. Freeze on the baking sheet for 15 minutes. (They can be placed quite close together, as they won't spread much while baking.)

Preheat oven to 350°F.

Bake the balls for 12–14 minutes.

Let your balls cool a little, then roll in the icing sugar. Let them cool completely and roll once more.

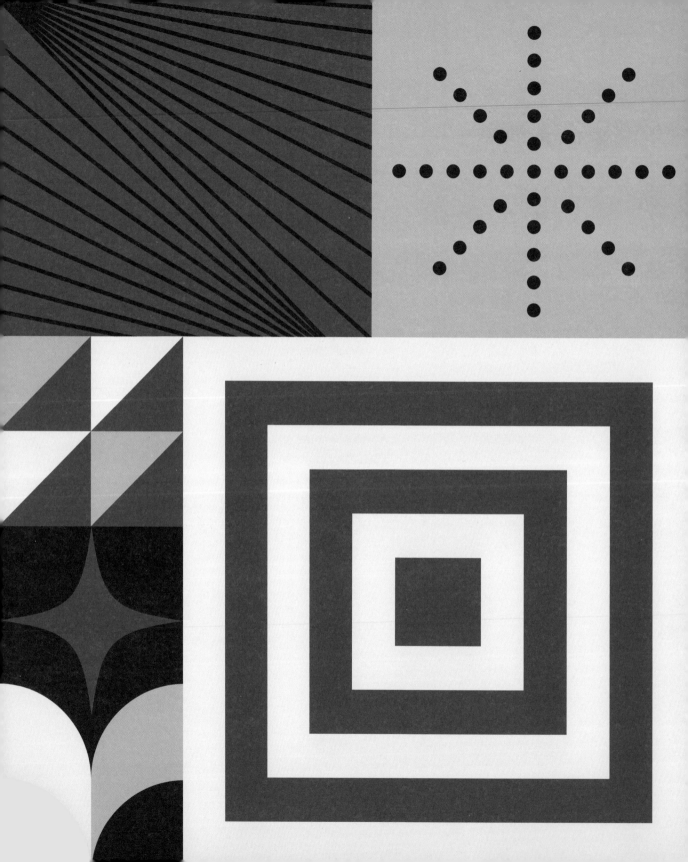

WEIRD
AND
WHIMSICAL

RECIPES

STORIES

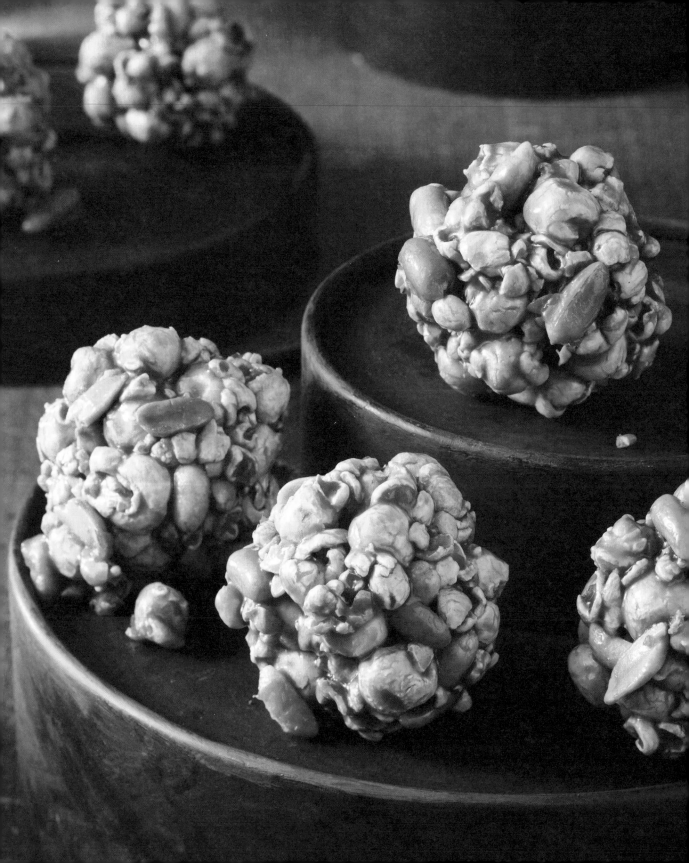

Baseball Caramel Corn Peanut Clusters

Easier than getting to first base.

Popcorn Kush is named for its compact, popcorn-shaped buds. Its description on one website made me laugh—apparently it pairs well with doing nothing.

Makes 20 popcorn balls with ½ cup cannabutter (just over 7 mg THC per ball).

7 cups of popped "movie theatre style" popcorn

½ cup (64 g) shelled, roasted, salted peanuts

1 cup (200 g) brown sugar

½ cup (125 mL) corn syrup

¼ cup (57 g) unsalted butter

½ tsp baking soda

½ cup (113 g) cannabutter, cut into small pieces

Line baking sheet(s) with parchment paper or silicone mat(s) and set aside. Toss the popcorn together with the peanuts in a large mixing bowl.

In a small saucepan over medium heat, stir together the brown sugar and corn syrup until the sugar melts. Clip on a candy thermometer and reduce the heat to medium-low.

Stir in the regular butter and the baking soda. Heat to between 235°F and 250°F, somewhere in the neighbourhood of "soft ball" to "firm ball," whisking regularly so that your mixture doesn't burn. (Make sure the little nub of your thermometer is down in there so you can regulate.) Double-check that you've hit the right heat by dropping a little caramel into cold water; it should turn into a wee softball.* If you've gotten it right, remove the caramel from the heat and add the cannabutter, whisking hard to fully incorporate.

Using a silicone spatula, pour the caramel over the popcorn and nuts in about three globs, folding the gooey in after each addition.

Let the caramel cool for a minute or so, and then form golf-ball-sized treats using your hands, setting them on the baking sheet(s) to cool completely.

*If you're not sure if the caramel is the right temp, and the caramel turned into candy when you added it to the cold water, toss it and start again! You really don't want to waste your cannabutter. (I may or may not have experienced this. At the photoshoot for this recipe.)

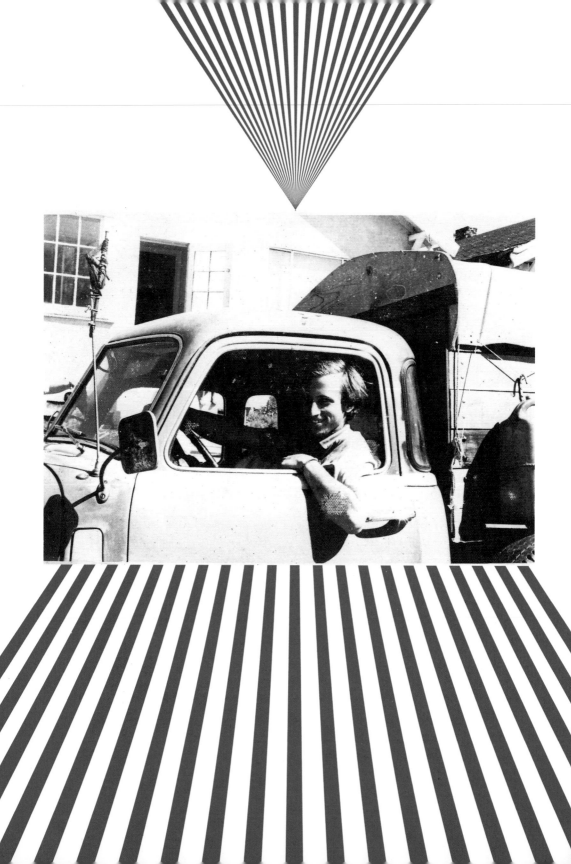

Jim Cooperman

Jim Cooperman is the author of *Everything Shuswap* and writes a blog focused on the geography of the Shuswap region in BC, shuswappassion.ca. His local environmental work led to the protection of over 25,000 hectares of new parks in the Shuswap, which is documented in the book *Big Trees Saved* by Deanna Kawatski. Jim lives with his wife, Kathleen, in a log home they built on forty acres above Shuswap Lake, where they raised their five children.

My interview with Jim takes a gently different format from the other interviews, as my GD phone recorder didn't work for our discussion. What do you want from a cannabis baker, you think we're perfect? Luckily I had taken careful notes, but because I hadn't captured Jim's exact words in all cases, I had to change the format to more of an article style. Jim edited the piece after we were finished, and it turned out beautifully, so all's well that ends well.

"There were only two options for me in 1969—prison or Canada," Jim tells me over the phone from his hand-built home across the country from me in the Shuswap in southern British Columbia, where he settled after escaping the Vietnam draft over fifty years ago. Jim was peace loving and passionately against the war, seeing it as illegal and immoral. He helped organize a 1967 anti-war demonstration at the Induction Center in Oakland, California, by cruising the streets with a loudspeaker, encouraging great crowds, before being forced back by waves of police descending with batons. The next day, Jim spoke to the crowd at Sproul Hall on the Berkeley campus, inspiring about 1,000 protestors to picket peacefully; a larger protest involving upwards of 10,000 activists took place at the end of the week, which resulted in the National Guard arriving to disperse the crowds.

"Those were crazy times," Jim says. "It was a mix of very serious activism, but we were also young, so it was a party, too. I remember attending the first Be-In, in Golden Gate Park with Allen Ginsberg, the Grateful Dead, and many other bands, and it was a fabulous time. If you want to read a good book about what things were like in the sixties, check out *Hippie*, by Barry Miles. There was lots of music and dancing; it was just such a party. Some of the activists didn't like that—they wrote articles saying that the hippies weren't taking things seriously enough. Because those two things don't mix, really, serious activism and having a good time. But I somehow managed to do both. I kept my grades up and graduated with a psychology degree after four years.

"When I graduated, though, that meant that my student deferment was gone, even though I went on to graduate school in San Francisco. The military was all over that campus, and classes were cancelled. It was nuts. I knew that time was running out."

Jim was called to the Induction Center where he had protested earlier, but this time, as a potential recruit, for a preinduction physical.

"I hid a pencil in my underwear," he said, "and I wrote on my papers *Get out of Vietnam*. The doctor saw what I had written and sent me to the commander's office.

"I confronted the officer, asking him, 'Where's your conscience? How can you send men off to kill and be killed in an illegal war?'

"He said that he was helping protect our freedoms and told me that the next time I was summoned it would be for induction. He was never able to fulfill that threat. Two weeks later I crossed the border into Canada."

Jim and his pregnant first wife loaded up their twenty-year-old truck and homemade camper, "Lucy," with two dogs, a cat, and some homesteading tools, and they headed north. A year after they settled, he wrote the poem "At the Border."

Here I stand head in hand
I turn my face to the green mountains
Leaving behind that land filled with
Electric, antiseptic multi-component opponents
A product of United States Foreign Policy
Unable to make it with those people
I despised their evil ways
War over there, everywhere

I asked how cannabis fit into his life as a hippie.

"Cannabis has always been part of my life as an adult, although I've never really 'come out' about it," Jim said. "Of course, it was illegal, so we always had to be careful. I learned recently that the government deliberately used it to imprison Black people and protestors. That's terrible, awful, but I didn't know it at the time.

"We used to get it in matchboxes for five dollars, and it was full of stems and seeds. And then because I always seemed to have a line on where to get some, I'd become kind of a mini dealer by purchasing kilos wrapped in cellophane and dividing it up for friends—just making enough to pay for my own supply. Later, where we lived in rural BC, there was a scarcity of pot, but we were able to grow sativa from Mexican pot seeds. Sativa grown outdoors doesn't reach maturity this far north, so we just smoked the tops that had the most THC. In the early eighties, indica came onto the scene, likely from Thai stick seeds. That was a huge change that improved the quality from 200 to 400 percent, when the smoking shifted to buds. Soon, people started growing under lights indoors to produce clones to plant in the bush, eliminating the need to plant seeds and having to wait for the males to show themselves, which was a game changer. Then people started growing plants indoors year-round, and within a few years, BC Bud had become famous. The bud available now is much stronger than what we grew outdoors in the eighties, although I can remember back at Berkeley lying on the floor listening to music and hallucinating."

And on its effects: "When you're a homesteader, there's a lot of work to be done, and cannabis keeps your mind occupied to avoid the monotony. It improves mood, creativity, imagination, and helps spark ideas. I can always get more done with writing and environmental action, too. But I rarely partook at meetings or actions, instead saving it as a treat for the evening break times.

"Almost everyone uses one type of drug or another. Alcohol, coffee, and cigarettes are the most common ones. Then there are all the prescription drugs, and there are even some religious activities that produce drug-like effects in the brain. Out of all of these, I think that cannabis is the best and least problematic; it's unlikely that people who are high get angry, cause violence, or engage in something nasty (of course, there are exceptions to every rule). Basically, THC elevates mood, enhances mindspace, and brings smiles. It goes well with music and dancing! But of course, it's certainly not for everyone. The key is moderation, avoiding the harder drugs, and not mixing drugs.

"Oh, and I always had a rule: No toking in the morning. I've always thought that morning time should be enhancement free, so that there's a difference in your day. I often saved jobs for the afternoon, when enhancement could take the boredom away.

"And no one should really be smoking over the age of sixty. I smoked a bit too long, and I'm paying for it now, by having to cope with mild asthma. Move on to edibles as early as you can, but each time, be sure to plan ahead for the prolonged effects.

"For me, THC has been helpful throughout my life. I use it in moderation and avoid all the other psychedelics. Over my seventy-five years, I've come up with many creative, unique ideas after some enhancement. Amazingly, many became reality. But everything began with the goal to live close to the land in rural BC with other like-minded people. And I'm not finished—I continue to write articles and commentaries, with Kathi's help, and produce more community music events, both in Salmon Arm and here on the North Shuswap."

You're a wise man, Jim, in many ways, especially when you're encouraging sensible use of edibles. Thanks for your peaceful perspective and many decades of environmental conservation work.

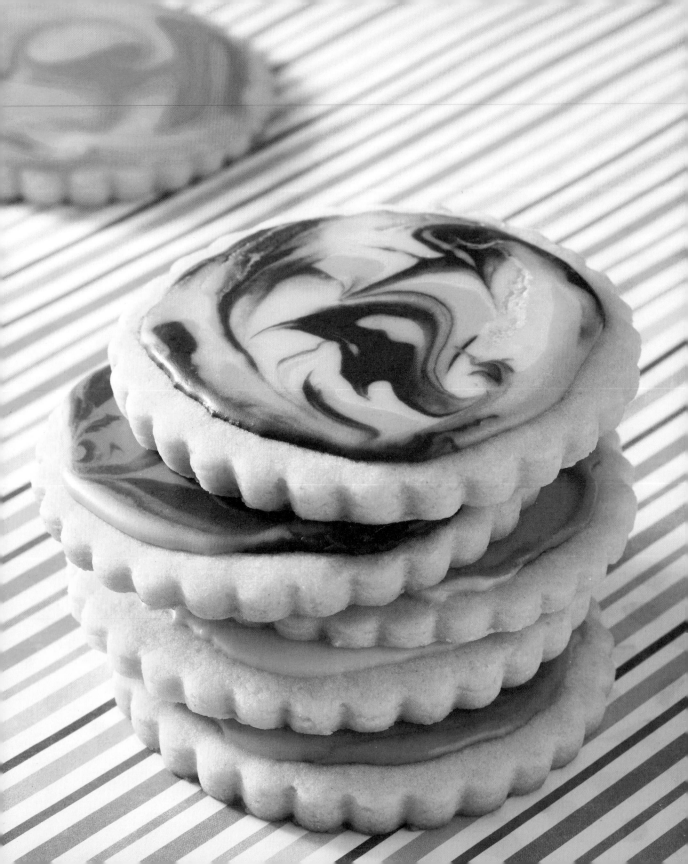

Tie-Dye Lemon Sugar Cookies

Making these is easier than waking up with a VW van's gear shift poking your back.

SUGGESTED MOOD/STRAIN

Hippie Crippler is a sativa-dominant hybrid that may offer that happy yet spaced-out feeling.

Makes 23 cookies with ½ cup cannabutter (about 6 mg THC per piece).

Cookies

½ cup (113 g) cannabutter

½ cup (113 g) unsalted butter, melted

1 cup (200 g) granulated sugar

1 egg

1 tsp lemon extract

1 tsp vanilla extract

1 lemon, zested, a quarter of the lemon juiced and reserved for the icing

3 cups (426 g) all-purpose flour

1 tsp baking powder

Dash of salt

Icing

5½ cups (622 g) icing (powdered) sugar + more if needed, sifted

7 Tbsp pasteurized egg whites, + more if needed*

1 tsp lemon extract

Tie-dye-style gel colours (at least 3)

To make the cookies: Melt the cannabutter in a double boiler or in a heat-proof bowl over a pot of simmering water.

With your favourite mixer, combine the butters with the sugar. Add in the egg, extracts, and zest.

In a separate bowl, stir together the flour, baking powder, and salt. Add to the mixing bowl in a few additions. Divide the dough in half, wrap both doughs with plastic wrap, and flatten them into discs. Refrigerate for at least 30 minutes.

Preheat the oven to 350°F and line baking sheet(s) with parchment paper or silicone mat(s). Roll out the dough to a one-quarter-inch thickness. Cut cookies with a 3½-inch round cookie cutter and place them on the baking sheet(s), with about an inch between each cookie. Ball up the dough, roll again, and cut more, taking breaks to chill the dough for a bit if it gets too soft to easily work with. Repeat with the remaining dough disc.

Bake for 8 minutes, trying not to brown the edges of the cookies. Cool on the baking sheets for 5–10 minutes before removing to a cooling rack. Let cookies cool completely before decorating.

To make the icing and to decorate the cookies: Wash that mixer, and combine the icing sugar and the egg whites. Add the lemon extract. Using a knife, cut into the icing—it should take 8 seconds to seal up that cut line. If slower than that, add some lemon juice; if faster, add icing sugar. Drive yourself mental flipping between the two for a while.

Separate the icing into small bowls. Stir in your gel colouring (one colour for each bowl) and cover with damp dishcloths until ready to use.

Set a baking sheet under the wire rack of cooled cookies. Dollop small spoonfuls of 3 colours onto a cookie. Don't be shy to cross one colour over the next, keeping a li'l finger bowl of water and a dry towel nearby. Now here's whatcher gonna do. Using a clean fingertip, gently swipe one colour into the next, breaking up the big globs. Dip into the finger bowl and do the next glob. Drag icing lumps toward the edges of the cookie. Repeat, making cute curls and swirls, not digging in too far. Now, take a skewer and draw lines within the swirls. Voila! Tie-dye! Repeat with the next cookie, and the one after that. It may take you a few tries to nail this, but the first ones will be appreciated just as much as the last.

Let the icing set for at least an hour, preferably overnight. Peace, dudes.

*Pasteurized egg whites: Buying these in a carton lets you skip the pasteurization step. If using regular eggs, see directions about how to pasteurize them on page 47.

Candied Maple Bacon Cheesecake Cookies

Easier than green eggs and ham (cookies).

Let's go with *Unicorn Bacon*,
a sativa-dominant THC strain.

Makes 24 cookies with ½ cup
cannabutter (about 6 mg THC
per cookie).

Candied Bacon*
1 lb (500 g) thick-cut bacon
½ cup (100 g) brown sugar
  + more if needed

Graham Cookies
½ cup (113 g) cannabutter
1 cup (227 g) unsalted butter, room
  temperature
½ cup (100 g) brown sugar
½ cup (100 g) granulated sugar
1 egg + 1 yolk
2¼ cups (355 g) all-purpose flour
1¾ cups (175 g) graham cracker
  crumbs, divided**
3 Tbsp cornstarch
Dash of salt

Cheesecake Filling
1 box (250 g; 9 oz) cream cheese,
  softened (microwave 15–20 seconds)
1 egg
¼ cup (63 mL) maple syrup
½ tsp maple extract

To make the candied bacon: Preheat oven to 350°F, and set
a rack over a baking sheet lined with foil. Lay the strips of
bacon flat across the rack.

Sprinkle the brown sugar evenly over the bacon, so that it
looks like an even layer of sand. (If you run a bit short, add
more as needed.)

Cook the bacon until crisp, for about 45 minutes
(checking regularly near the end so that it doesn't burn).
No need to flip. When cool enough to handle, dice the
deliciousness. Go ahead and snack on some of that bacon. It's
amazing.

To make the graham cookies and cheesecake filling: While the
bacon is cooking, melt the cannabutter in a double boiler or
in a heat-proof bowl over a pot of simmering water. Use your
favourite mixer to combine the butters and sugars. Add the
egg and yolk.

In a separate bowl, using a wooden spoon, mix together
the flour, 1¼ cups graham crumbs, cornstarch, and salt. Add
to the mixing bowl in a few additions. Put the dough into the
fridge to chill for a few minutes.

Prepare another baking sheet, this time with parchment
paper or a silicone mat. Roll generous 1½-Tbsp cookie scoops
of dough into balls, roll the balls in the ½ cup of reserved
graham cracker crumbs, and space the balls at least an inch
apart on the baking sheet. Chill for at least 30 minutes.

Meanwhile, wash the bowl of your mixer. Combine
softened cream cheese, egg, maple syrup, and maple extract
until very smooth.

For the big finish: Preheat oven to 350°F (again). Make
indentations in the centre of each cookie using a wine cork or

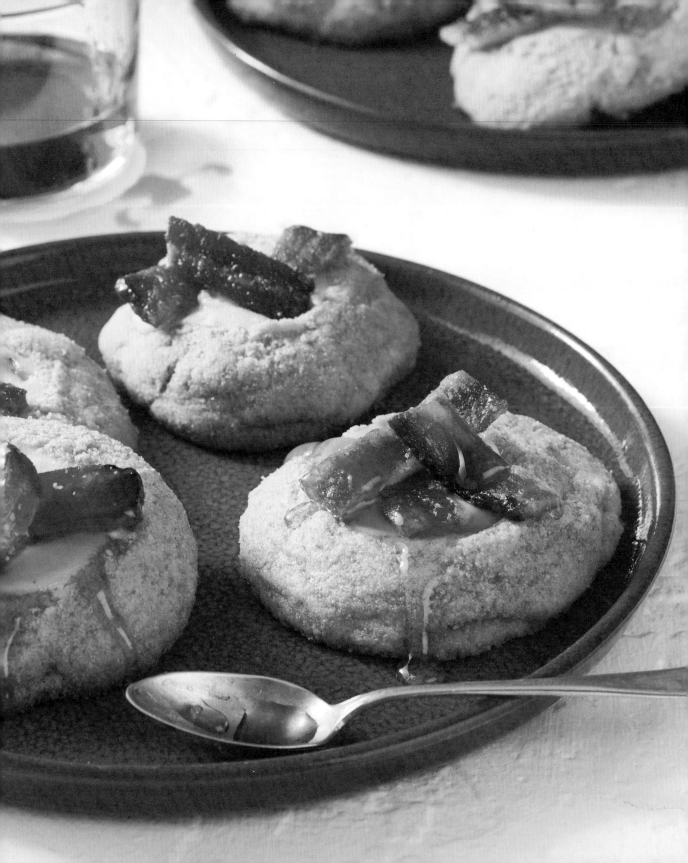

screw top (i.e., a washed lid of an olive oil bottle or similar). Spoon filling into the divot of each cookie. Bake for about 10 minutes, until the edges of the cookies just begin to brown and the cheese is gently firm.

Let the cookies rest for about 5 minutes before removing to a cooling rack. Top with the candied bacon, if you haven't already eaten it all. Repeat, using all dough. Drizzle with a hint more maple syrup if you want to double down on the Canadiana.

*Veggies can omit the candied bacon and top with any traditional fruity cheesecake topping.

**Graham cracker crumbs: Buy these, or use a food processor to pulse the whole crackers.

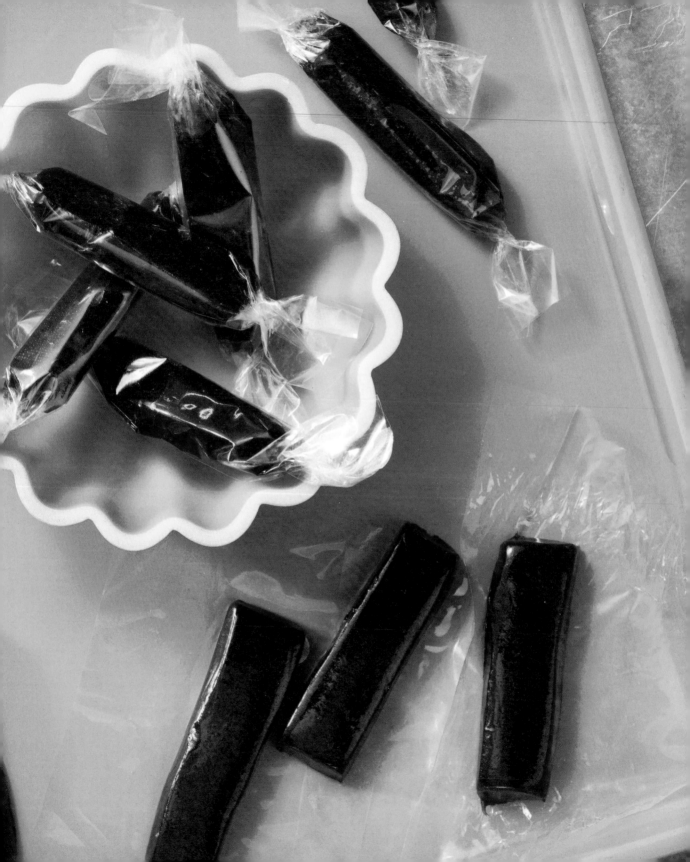

Black Licorice Toffees

This recipe is easier than smiling with black teeth.

SUGGESTED MOOD/STRAIN

Licorice Kush is an indica-dominant strain that is uplifting and calming, good for depression and mood. Be careful if you find some, though—it's high in THC.

Makes about 40 toffees with ½ cup cannabutter (over 3 mg THC per piece). You can handle a couple.

½ cup (113 g) cannabutter
1 cup (200 g) granulated sugar
A scant cup (200 mL; 7 oz) sweetened condensed milk
¾ cups (188 mL) corn syrup
¼ cup (63 mL) cooking molasses*
1 tsp anise or star anise extract
Black gel colouring

Prepare a 9 × 9–inch pan, spraying with non-stick cooking spray, then lining it with parchment paper; make two 9 × 14–inch parchment strips. Criss-cross the strips into the pan, hanging them over the sides. If you only have an 8 × 8–inch pan you're fine, just compensate by slicing thinner strips of toffee in the end, as your candy will be thicker in the pan.

Add all ingredients except the anise extract and gel colouring to a medium saucepan, and clip on your candy thermometer. Give all a stir with a wooden spoon for a while, and then switch over to a whisk.

When your witches' brew begins to bubble, you really don't need to stir it much anymore; just keep an eye on your candy thermometer (make sure its li'l nub is submerged). When it hits 246°F, remove from heat, and whisk in the anise extract. Next add in a few drops of the black gel colouring, stirring and adding more until you get a lovely midnight colour.

Pour your toffee into the prepared pan. Let it cool on the counter until just warm, and then pop it into the fridge until cold and solid.

Use a heavy knife to slice the block of toffee away from the edge of the pan, using the handles to lift it onto the counter. Remove the parchment. Cut the block into strips, and then squares and rectangles. Don't stress about the exact shape yet, but try to get them to be around the same weight per piece.

Cut rectangles of wax paper (or cellophane) big enough to wrap your licorice pieces. As you wrap, you can mould the toffee into longer rectangle shapes, keeping the paper between your fingers and the toffee so that your minging fingerprints aren't all over people's treats.

Drop all tools into water immediately to soak, to avoid sticky situations.

*It's important to use cooking molasses for this recipe, as it's stronger than fancy molasses.

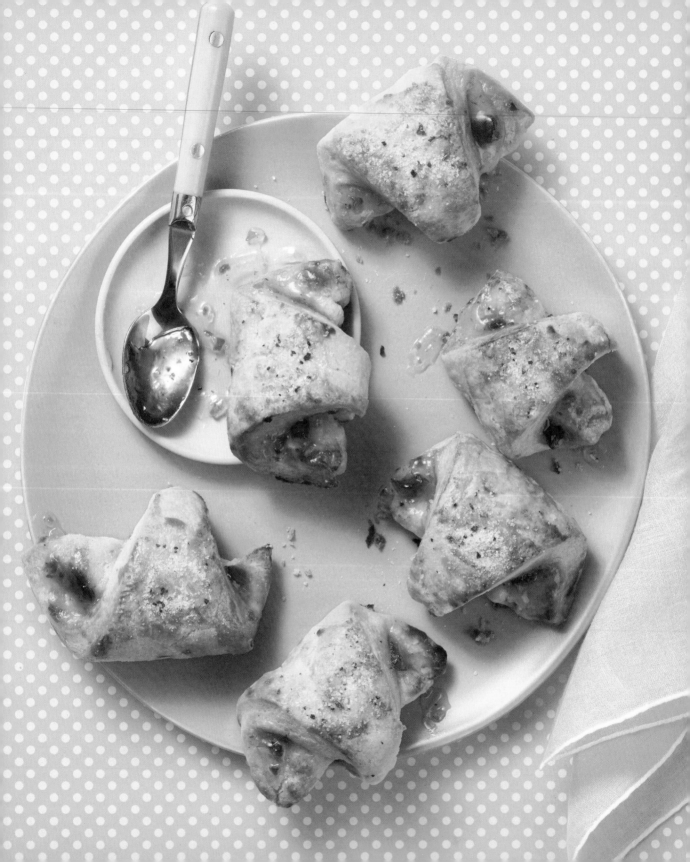

Jalapeño Jelly Rugelach with Truffle Salt

Making these is easier than being a truffle pig. (I think. Maybe they actually have a lot of fun.)

SUGGESTED MOOD/STRAIN
Kosher Dawg is a hybrid strain giving feelings of calm and a desire to find a blanket.

Makes 32 rugelach with ½ cup cannabutter (almost 5 mg THC per piece). This recipe combines favourites of one friend who loves this decadent pastry (derived from the Jewish communities of Poland) and another who loves truffle. The "weird and whimsical" bit is combining these flavours, and with a bit of sweet and spice, too.

2 cups (284 g) all-purpose flour
½ tsp salt
½ cup (113 g) cold or frozen cannabutter, cubed
½ cup (113 g) cold unsalted butter, cubed
1 box (250 g; 8 oz) cold cream cheese, cubed
1 egg yolk + 1 additional egg reserved for egg wash
About half a small jar of jalapeño jelly
A few pinches of truffle salt*

Prep baking sheet(s) with parchment or silicone mat(s). In the bowl of your food processor (or on a pastry board with two criss-cross Edward Scissorhands knives going), combine the flour with the salt, adding in the butters and cream cheese, pulsing (or cutting in) until you get a grainy consistency. Add the egg yolk and the dough should come together. Divide into 4 equal parts. Refrigerate whichever dough lumps you aren't currently working with.

Smooth one of the lumps into a ball. Spread more parchment over a work surface and roll the dough out onto it into a circle about ¼-inch thick. Slice the circle into 8 equal parts, kind of like a pizza.

With a pastry brush, spread the jalapeño jelly across the surface of the circle. Starting at the rounded edge of a "pie slice," roll inward, tucking the point beneath the rugelach. Place the roll on the baking sheet. Repeat with all triangles, and then with all dough.

Wash your brush, whisk the reserved egg in a small bowl, and give the rugelach an egg wash. Sprinkle with truffle salt. Refrigerate all for about an hour.

Preheat oven to 350°F. Cook the rugelach until gently browned, 25–30 minutes.

*Truffle salt can be found in most snobby grocery stores. I apologize that it's a bit spendy, but once you have it, there will be no shortage of ways to use it.

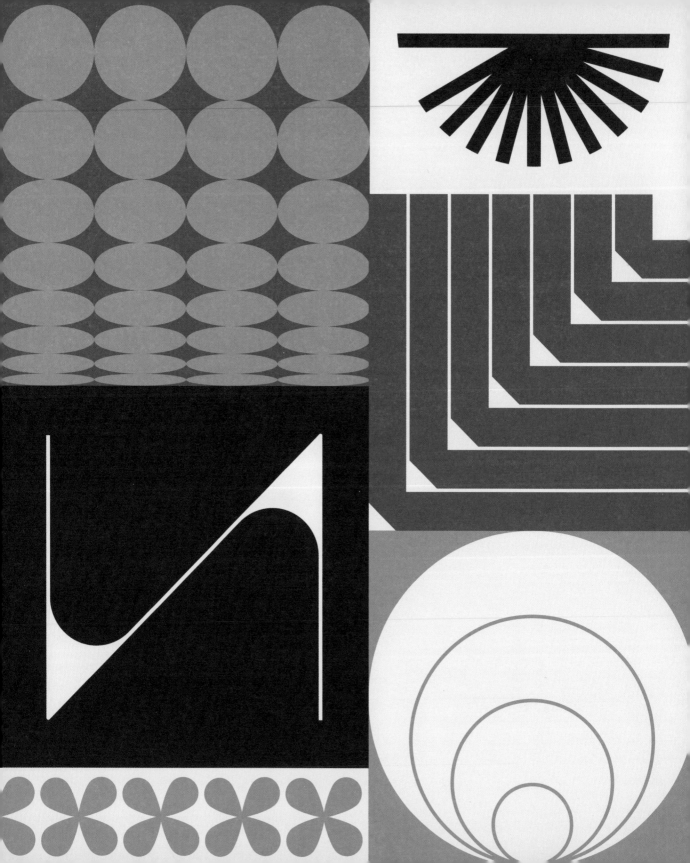

SAVOURIES

RECITES

STORIES

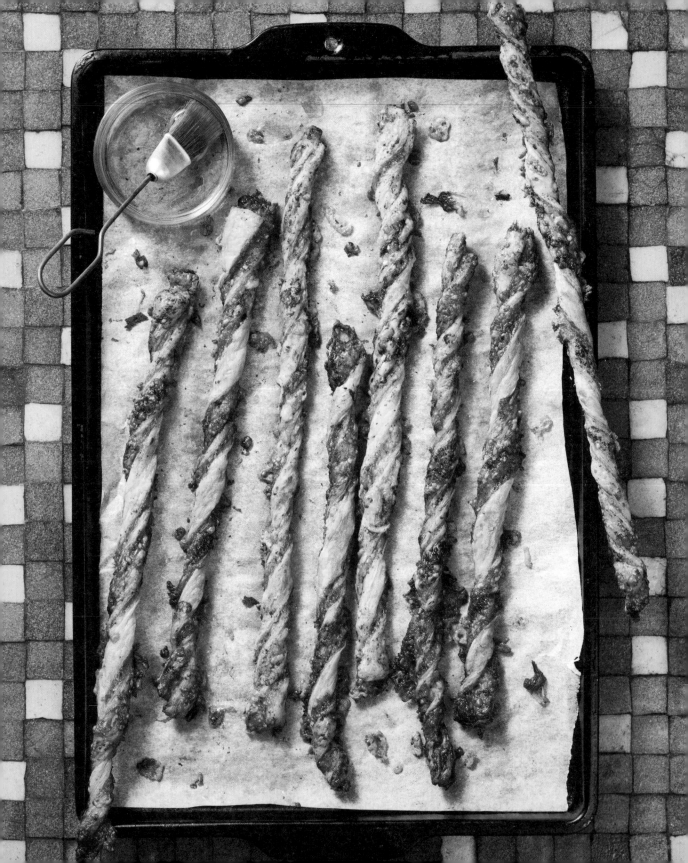

Cheesy Breadstick Twists with Black Olive Tapenade

Making these is easier than drinking through a cheese straw.

Makes 32 cheese twists with 5 Tbsp cannavirgin olive oil (almost 4 mg THC per 2 twists)

1 package (450 g) frozen puff pastry, thawed*

1 egg

¼ cup (60 g) puréed pitted black olives or store-bought tapenade

5 Tbsp cannavirgin olive oil

1 cup (113 g) old cheddar cheese, grated, packed

1 cup (85 g) Parmesan, grated, packed

Preheat oven to 375°F. Sandwiched between sheets of parchment paper, roll out one of the puff pastry rectangles as thin as you can get it. Slice off any weird edges and toss the excess.

In a small bowl, whisk the egg. Brush the pastry with egg wash. In another small bowl, add the infused oil to the tapenade.

In yet another small bowl, toss the cheeses together. Sprinkle half of the tapenade over the pastry, followed by the cheese.

Repeat your parchment-sandwich-rolling deal with the other sheet of pastry. Lay this pastry atop the first cheesy one. Trim the edges and toss so that you're working with a perfect rectangle, and lift the parchment directly onto a baking sheet.

Repeat the egg wash, tapenade spread, and cheesy sprinkle overtop, using up all remaining ingredients. (Except maybe the rest of the egg. Who cares?)

Using a sharp knife, slice the large pastry rectangle in half width-wise, and go at each rectangle, slicing in half in the same direction again into 4 long pieces. Now carefully cut each piece into quarters, again in the same direction, until we get to pieces about ¼-inch wide. Don't stress about exact numbers here, just try to nail something you can work with.

Preheat the oven to 375°F. Twist your first pastry strip into some twirls, pressing the ends down to secure. Repeat with all remaining pastry strips. Can I say strip more often? I think I can. Toss ingredients that fell off over the tops of the strips. (Told you!)

Bake your strips (boom) until golden brown, about 25 minutes. These will be a bit long to manage in terms of snacking, so feel free to slice again to serve, just be sure to somehow eat enough to get a solid dose. (I have faith in you.)

*Frozen puff pastry: Comes as 2 sheets. Thaw overnight in the fridge, if you can remember. Do not thaw in microwave. It will get mushy.

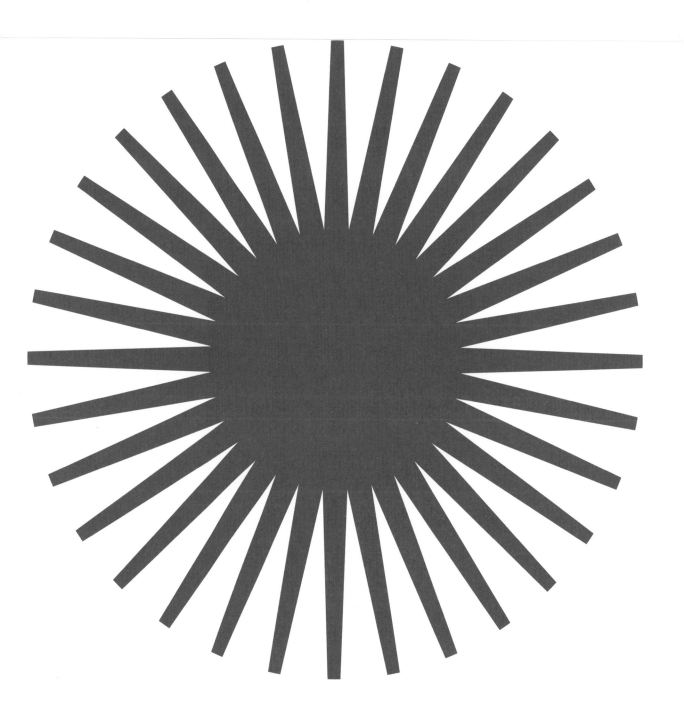

Chas

Chas is a veteran of the U.S. Marines, who served in Iraq. He's currently a teacher based in San Diego and an amateur grower. We met through Instagram. Chas has chosen not to share his last name or photo because he works with young people and is concerned that, sadly, there still might be judgement among their parents.

I think I tried cannabis maybe twice in high school. And not with any really amazing results either. Actually, the first time I tried cannabis I got busted by my parents. They found some paraphernalia in my bag, and then it was like, okay, great, well this is over. After that, I really kind of turned it off until college; then, I wouldn't say that it was a positive experience or a negative experience, but it definitely wasn't an enriching experience, if that makes sense. I ended up falling away from it for a long time, especially with going into the military.

I joined the Marine Corps in 1999. I went to boot camp in '99, and, you know, obviously, you have to abstain from cannabis when you're in the military. I think you still have to do that . . . Actually, I don't know if that's true or not.

What inspired me to enlist? You know, this was before 9/11, so enlisting wasn't this whole patriotic thing—not for me then, anyway. It was more that I knew I was a great athlete, great at learning through my hands, great at doing things, and that school

then wasn't really my strength. So it was just like, okay, what can I do that's going to help me out with school when I'm ready? I wanted to better myself, while doing the full hands-on, but also contribute to the greater good. And I do think there was a part of me that thought, "Yeah, I can defend my country!" [*Chas laughs.*] And as a younger person—and not just younger, but before I had had the experience of being deployed—joining the military was pretty easy to do. If I could just set aside the political ramifications, the humanitarian ramifications, the personal and ethical ramifications, I think . . . I shouldn't say it was easy, exactly, but for me it was a good fit. It was very physically demanding; you follow directions, support one another, enter a brotherhood . . . it made a lot of sense.

I got deployed in 2004 to what was considered OIF2 [*Operation Iraqi Freedom II*]. I left for Iraq in August '04 and came back in April '05. I was a combat engineer attached to the infantry unit. It was a pretty intense and traumatic deployment. We were over there at a time that was supposed to be somewhat humanitarian. Saddam had been ousted, so we were supposed to be going over to do more training with the Iraqi police and Iraqi National Guard, which we did, daily, but still, we were taking anywhere between ten and fifteen enemy attacks a day on our battalion, most of those being indirect fire—RPGs [*rocket-propelled grenades*], rockets, and car bombs, but you know, there were also several instances where an IED [*improvised explosive device*] or blast would be associated with an ambush. We went in and kind of took over two small, pretty hostile towns, and lived in and occupied those for a little while.

We'd do vehicle patrols down canal roads or to somewhere, and then we'd give out foot patrol with our mine detectors and search for large weapons caches. When we were in-country, it wasn't like we were fighting an enemy that had giant artillery cannons. I mean, sure, there were rockets, RPGs, rocket launchers, things like that, but there were also 250-pound and 500-pound bombs everywhere. They had no means to deploy them, except by burying them or hiding them as these giant roadside bombs or IEDs. So one of our primary roles was to cordon off areas, searching the houses and the land to look for large weapons caches. Which we found. I mean . . . just hundreds of thousands of pounds of weapons. The first weapons cache we found was ten 500-pound bombs. And then we'd just use a good amount of C-4, detonate in place, and move on with our day, just to get rid of them. So I mean, there were lots of explosions, lots of indirect and direct blasts, with some of our shots like "How close can we stay to this one?"—kind of being a little silly in-country.

I took a blast injury in late November of 2004 that disabled my truck. We drove around then in pretty unarmored vehicles—open window, quarter-inch steel—so you know, shrapnel just kind of went through them. Our equipment saved our lives, but our vehicle was disabled. We took a pretty big blast, but we all walked away somehow.

But I think that over there it wasn't super traumatic.

The more I learn about myself and think about it, it was almost like caveman brain, or the most primitive brain turned on. All you're worried about over there is survival. Like, you have an MRE [meal,

ready to eat]—it's not great food, but you've got food, you have water in your truck . . . All you really have to do is take care of your guys, the eight or twelve or however many Marines are around you. And you kind of knew that if you walked out the gate to this base, and you died, or your buddy died, it was nothing you did. You could have been doing everything right. So it really was like okay, let's see what today holds, let's hope we get to dinner tonight, or chow, or wherever we ended up for our meal, in someone's home that we posted up in for the night, or our small outpost, or at one of our forward operating bases. Yeah, it was really easy over there. I mean, it sounds crazy, but I didn't have to worry about the balance in my bank account, getting fired, maintaining a job, health care, or my retirement.

But there was also a lot I didn't realize until later.

I mean, even just this year, I acknowledged to myself how much fear I lived in every minute of every day. If I had had this interview with you probably even six months ago, and you had asked, "Hey, were you afraid in Iraq?" I'd have said, "Well, no. Yes, we had to respond, and there was startle stuff." But then when you really think about it—leaving the base, knowing there's literally a cross hair, whether physically or figuratively on your head, knowing that someone is trying to kill you or your convoy, the people around you . . . of course, there's just this amazing fear of death surrounding you.

How was coming back? I mean, the gates of hell come to mind. The first two or three years back were especially hard. Coming back initially, for the first two, three, maybe six months, there's almost this extreme high, like "I can get in my own car, not strap down my gear, and I don't have a rifle on me," which at one point, you feel kind of naked, but you're also like "Okay, this is good, I can put my arm out my window and it's not going to get blown off," things like that. But then, even though you think those fears are gone, none of it has actually gone away. If there's an animal carcass on the road, and you're driving with your partner, all of a sudden you freak out. There's a pretty visceral reaction and response to "I'm not safe, I'm in harm's way." Lots of those quick startles were really evident for me in those first few years back.

And I don't know if it was my medicine choice or not, but I definitely drank. Not every night, but I drank to black out, to a very, very dark spot. Drinking is definitely a depressant, and it exacerbated all of those emotions, feelings, responses that were within me. For that reason, I've chosen not to have a drink since 2007. But up to that point, and even moving past that, everything was pretty dark, scary, and overwhelming. I mean, just walking down the block in Baltimore, among the high-rise buildings, reminded me of patrolling cities that had two- and three-storey buildings that were very heavily occupied. I didn't trust any car that was loaded with people, or anyone who was driving quickly toward me. I didn't trust anyone who was up on a balcony or anywhere above me. So yeah, even just parking my car at night and walking back to my building elevated my nervous system response. I only realized how much those feelings affected every minute of every day later.

And then that's where my cannabis journey started, a little bit. Cannabis was still very taboo then. It wasn't really associated with being medicinal, at least in the community I was part of at the time. Being on the East Coast, in Baltimore, even veterans weren't really connected. I did reach out to a buddy, though, got some, and ended up smoking it occasionally. I'm very sensitive to THC and cannabinoids, so even a small amount can really hit me, and there was definitely paranoia and anxiety

involved. But I found that after the initial ninety minutes wore off, I was in a space that was very hard for me to get to on my own. I got relaxed—comfortable. Cannabis was physically and emotionally soothing to my nervous system. So to me, that kind of pointed out, "Okay, there's something going on here, and there has to be a way that I can get those benefits in the end phase to happen earlier."

After I stopped drinking at first, I did kind of adopt an abstinence-only type idea. That brought some internal conflict when I finally reached back for cannabis's medicine. The big question for me was whether this substance was enriching my life, or whether it was taking something away. I started to see that unlike alcohol, cannabis was having a very positive effect. And then jump to 2012—I had major hip surgery. I had some congenital stuff going on, but had also always struggled with the effects of being deployed, sitting at end range with my full load on, doing foot patrols, vehicle patrols . . . My body felt awful. At first I just assumed, "Oh, once I'm away from a combat zone I'll feel better." I never felt better.

But if you can believe it, after the hip surgery, I came out of the hospital and never took another narcotic. I was bed bound for eight weeks. I became a very layman baker and made chocolate chip cookies out of cannabis-infused olive oil, and never, ever had to take a pill. And I was like, "Hold *on!*" That sold me. I really got to wondering what this medicine was that I was putting into my oil cookies. How was it grown? What was in it? And that jumped me into learning to grow my own medicine.

Now, I'm in San Diego, and statewide, we're allowed to have six plants. Which is kind of crazy, because that could be six scrawny, puny, ridiculous runts, or it could be six giant, ten-pound plants. But I like growing because I really like the idea of sustainability. I like to grow outdoors; I can literally grow year-round in a greenhouse because I choose to use autoflower plants as opposed to photoperiod plants, for the most part. I love the short stature of autoflower, and I love that I can go seed to harvest in sixty-five to one hundred days. I can do a continual harvest by popping, you know, four, five, or six seeds every month or two, and then every month or two, I'm harvesting a few plants, processing an oil, or processing a salve or tincture. Yeah, that's kind of become my model for my grow.

I have a friend who's a breeder in Maine, and he has a really nice two-parts CBD, one-part THC that I've been enjoying. That's been really nice for tincture; it helps me at night, with the noises that startle me, turning on my body to where I can't go back to sleep. And then the pain issues with the hip, the back, neck . . . cannabis is just great for the bodily issues. I like the discrete nature of the tincture. Not that I think there's anything inherently wrong with smoking, I mean, I don't think it can cause detrimental effects, but I try to do what I can athletically, and I value my lung response and reaction. I find that the high THC strains are the best for topical. I mean, CBD might work great for some people, but I don't know, for pain management and aches and pains, I find that high THC is best.

I think for me, cannabis isn't the best daytime medication for going to work, or I haven't found it to be. Most strains make me somewhat sleepy, a little bit groggy, so they work best at night. But I truly believe that, just in general, getting a good night's sleep and being pain-free are probably two of the best things you can do to promote your mental health. In the early days, the cookies delivered that support, but now I mostly rely on tincture, as I said.

And I've always refused the VA cocktail. Because it's like, "Great, I can get on the VA cocktail where I'm taking thirteen medications and I'm still suicidal?" Or I can not be on the medications and still be suicidal, like, what's the bonus? So I've chosen not to be on the cocktail. We all have our ebbs and flows in life, but I think learning to manage them, deal with them, and sit with them is really important as well.

I will say that overall . . . those "dark gates of hell" that I mentioned were the catalysts to my own spiritual journey—being open to meditation, being open to self-reflection, being open to learning more and listening to my body, and yeah, just listening and learning. I've connected with a really cool veterans' community on Instagram that is into regenerative agriculture, sustainable living, a little bit of spirituality—more of an overall healthy lifestyle.

Also, we've been hearing a lot over the past two years about psychedelic medicine. I've grown and used some over the past two, three, four months, and yeah, I think that's where that acknowledgement of fear I mentioned came from. It was like, hold on, this is exactly what I've been experiencing that has been affecting my life. It's pretty profound, the research and the results they're having with alternative therapies like psilocybin right now. What those seem to do, especially what they're noticing with depression, anxiety, and PTSD, is that they really hush the "default mode network." That's the network in your brain—kind of like, if you go sleigh riding, those sled trails that are constantly ingrained, that you can't get out of. Psilocybin seems to do a really good job of disrupting that.

I mean, honestly, cannabis has been the gateway to gardening, growing my own food, to learning about my soil microbes, learning how I can grow better plants and vegetables, to connecting with community members, and sharing information. I think if I hadn't been part of that small community from this plant, I don't think I would have considered exploring this new potentially beneficial style of medication. It's opened these little doors into thought processes that I might not have known I was open to. And I'm sure it's all the steps that I've taken, not just one.

I think that by having these conversations with our family, with our friends, about cannabis being an option—it's only going to continue to push the research field so that we really have a better understanding of "What cannabinoid is it that does this," or, "Hey, I have this cancer, how is it going to help?" So yeah, I just think that breaking the stigma, having these conversations, pushing them more, is the thing we need to do.

The last thing I would say is that my partner, my wife, she's never used cannabis in her life. She was somewhat apprehensive. But I think for her, truly seeing a plant go from the seed to this usable medicine has changed her viewpoint. I believe that watching this plant grow can change people's lives. It puts it in perspective that "Oh, hold on, we're demonizing this plant that we can all grow, and relate to, and connect with, and nurture." Yeah, I would encourage everyone to grow their own cannabis. Sure, we could all grow better cannabis, if we're not doing it professionally. But cannabis that's my own, that I've grown, that I've loved, has given me everything that I need, so I don't know that I ever need to not do that.

You know?

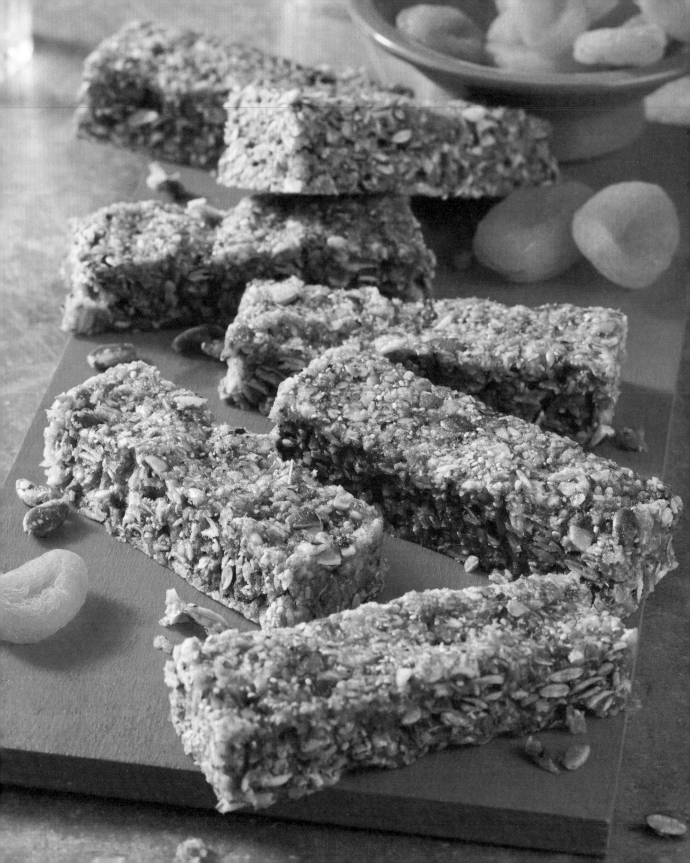

Seedy Bars

This recipe is easier than being a hungry vegan in a seedy bar. (I guess there are always fries.) I tried to get as many healthy descriptors into these bars as I could as penance for many of the other "less healthy, yet delicious" recipes here. So, these here bars are vegan, gluten-free, cold-pressed (because they were cold when I pressed them into their pan), caveman-friendly, and processed-sugar free. I'm also proud that these are nut-free, because we have allergies in our house, and I know that escaping nuts can sometimes be difficult.

SUGGESTED MOOD/STRAIN

Pumpkin Kush is an uplifting sativa-leaning hybrid.

Makes 12 bars with ¼ cup cannacoconut oil (almost 4 mg THC per piece).

1 cup (225 g) pitted dates
1 cup (225 g) dried (organic) apricots
¼ cup (57 g) cannacoconut oil
3 Tbsp pumpkin or sesame seed (tahini) butter
1 cup (90 g) unsweetened shredded coconut
1 cup (108 g) roasted, salted pepitas*
½ cup (67 g) salted sunflower seeds
¼ cup (40 g) hemp hearts
2 Tbsp chia seeds
2 Tbsp flax seeds

Soak the dates and apricots in hot water for 10 minutes. Drain 'em.

Melt the cannacoconut oil in a double-boiler or in a heat-proof bowl over a pot of simmering water.

In a food processor, turn your dates/apricots pasty. Add in the cannacoconut oil and the seed butter. Remove to your favourite mixer.

Add in the remaining ingredients and mix well.

Press the seedy dough into an 8 × 8–inch pan lined with parchment paper overhanging two sides. Chill for at least half an hour in the fridge. Lift the slab using the parchment handles, remove the paper, bisect the slab, and then divide both slabs lengthwise into 6 bars each.

*Roasted, salted pepitas (pumpkin seeds): I was lucky enough to buy them this way—try your fave bulk store. Otherwise, toss them with olive oil and salt and roast them on a baking sheet at 325°F for about 15 minutes.

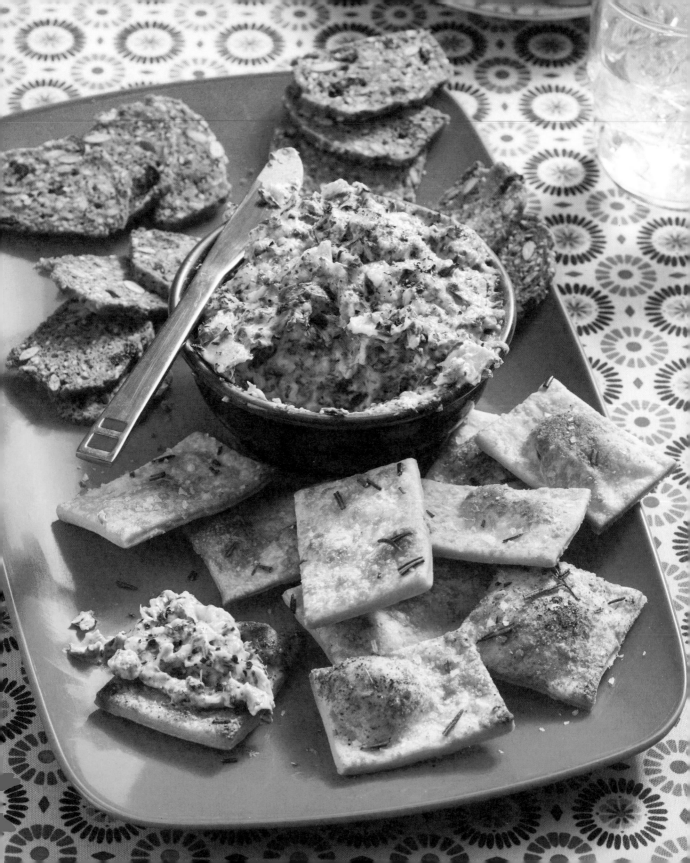

Cranberry Wheaten Toasts with Spinach Artichoke Jalapeño Dip

This recipe is easier than discussing Irish politics while stoned (or sober). My husband's family is from Northern Ireland, and a bread called "wheaten," that tastes like whole wheat banana-free banana bread, is always on the table there. These toasts taste similar, and they're even better slathered in homemade spinach artichoke dip.

SUGGESTED MOOD/STRAIN

Pot of Gold seems like a good strain for an Ireland-inspired recipe.

Makes 60 toasts with ¼ cup infused olive oil (about 1 mg THC per piece).

Toasts

½ cup (70 g) bread flour or all-purpose flour

½ cup (78 g) whole wheat flour

1 tsp baking soda

1 tsp coarse salt

½ cup (76 g) sesame seeds

⅓ cup (36 g) pepitas

¼ cup (36 g) cranberries, dried

1 Tbsp poppyseeds

A few pinches of fresh thyme

¾ cup (188 mL) buttermilk

¼ cup (63 mL) infused extra-virgin olive oil

Spinach Artichoke Dip

½ box (150 g) frozen spinach, thawed and drained

½ box (125 g; 4 oz) light cream cheese

½ cup (125 mL) onion-flavoured sour cream dip

½ cup (138 g) canned artichoke hearts, chopped

⅓ cup (28 g) Asiago cheese, shredded

⅓ cup (38 g) mozzarella cheese, shredded

2 Tbsp diced pickled jalapeños

Salt and pepper to taste

To make the toasts: Preheat oven to 350°F. In a medium mixing bowl, use a wooden spoon to combine the dry ingredients. Stir in the buttermilk and infused olive oil.

Spray down a squares pan (see page 22), and then press the dough into 6 of the square sections (a 9 × 5–inch loaf pan will also work). Bake for about 25 minutes, until a tester comes away clean. Allow the squares/loaf to cool, and then place in a plastic zipper bag and freeze until very solid, ideally overnight.

Preheat oven to 300°F. Using a very sharp, slim, unserrated knife, slice each square very thin. (I was able to get about 10 crackers out of each square.) If using a loaf pan, slice thin and then slice again into squares.

Spread the crackers on a baking sheet. Bake for about 15 minutes, flip each cracker, and bake for 5 minutes more, until all sides are gently browned.

To make the dip: Let the spinach thaw, and then squeeze all water out through a layer of cheesecloth (or a fine sieve, but that won't work quite as well). Otherwise, there's no magic here. Combine all ingredients in an oven-safe dish.

Before serving, preheat oven to 350°F. Bake dip for about 15 minutes, until the cheese is melted and gooey.

Serve warm with toasts.

Spinach Artichoke Jalapeño Dip shown with Cranberry Wheaten Toasts (back) and with Rosemary Garlic Sea-Salt Crackers (front, recipe on page 215)

Scott Milton

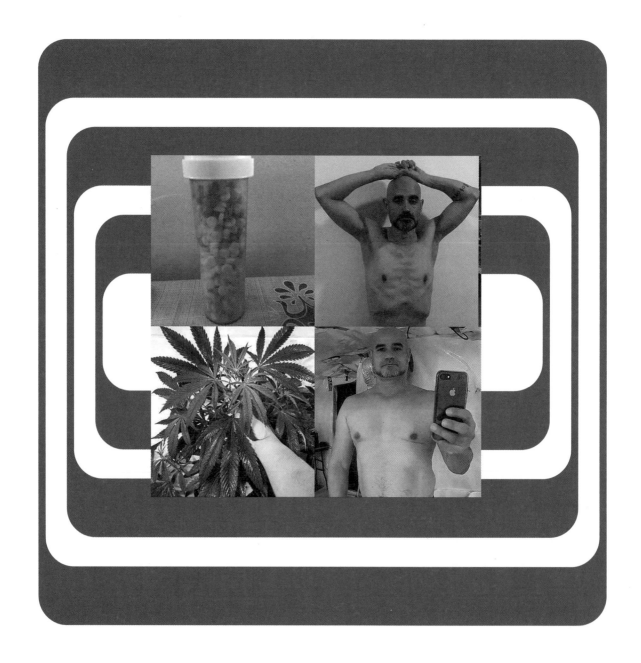

Scott Milton is a motivational speaker and cannabis grower who lives in Wheatland County, Alberta. I met Scott when, on Instagram, I saw the same before/after photo you're looking at right now. I was intrigued, and his story didn't disappoint.

I was born with epilepsy. My family has genetic epilepsy. It's crazy. We've lost two family members to the disease. My uncle, who—the British called it "having a fit," so actually, his death certificate says he fell off a cruise ship off the coast of India having a fit—he fell into the water and drowned. Plus, my twelve-year-old cousin, she had a seizure in the bathtub, and also drowned.

Epilepsy was classified as a mental health illness up until 1990, if you can believe it.

For me, living with this illness has been a journey. I've been in hospital so many times, hooked up to machines, for two and three weeks at a time. Not great. And in school, as a child, most of the seizures you're dealing with, the teacher thinks you're daydreaming. You kind of wander off, and can be gone not just for seconds, but for several minutes. I was actually targeted by one of my teachers when I was five years old—I mean, we're talking I was five in 1978. So the teacher actually started belting me across the back of the head, trying to get me to concentrate. That's how it was back then. But I told my mother, and that didn't turn out very well. My parents were military personnel, so . . . when parents arrive and find out their kid is being assaulted because he has seizures? Yeah, that was trouble.

But mainly, going through school, the seizures were very sporadic. It's when you get older that your environmental conditions can drive things. The seizures can actually go away . . . you might not even

have another one after your teenage years. Or, as they did with me, they can continue on, progressively getting worse, until you have a big seizure, which is a grand mal seizure. And then you collapse, and then they find out that . . . yup, that's what's going on. The big ones can get you locked into staying home a lot. You don't want to go out in public, so you start being a bit of a recluse and staying put. But I just forced myself out the door, not caring what happened. I just kept living my life the most I could back then.

My family and I have worked with the Alberta Children's Hospital and many of the Alberta Health Services for a long time. We've done our DNA profiles, and they've found a few things in there that have intrigued them. But what intrigues them quite a bit is also my transformation from using prescription drugs for many, many years to using cannabis instead.

[Here's an Ann intrusion for you so that you can catch on to where Scott is coming from more quickly than I did. I met Scott through Instagram, so I wasn't aware of his history at first. He spoke about substituting cannabis for "prescription drugs," and I assumed he was talking about opioids, which is a therapeutic avenue I'd heard many have had success with. In Scott's case, though, he was talking about substituting cannabis for his epilepsy drugs.]

Most of the drugs that are out there, ironically enough, the ones that are available, are not even specifically for epilepsy; one is called Dilantin, and the other is called carbamazepine, which is Tegratol. These drugs are actually used for schizophrenia and shell-shock victims, from wars, when they shake all the time, but they started experimenting on people with epilepsy with them. Some of the drugs were first synthesized in the thirties, that's how old they are. And they, of course, have terrible side effects. My side effects were piling one on top of the other because I was taking five different medications. If you had seen how many pills I was taking a day, it was probably about thirty. And I was still having 400 seizures per month.

In my pictures, you can see the effects. When I was on all those drugs, I was left with about 118 pounds of bone and skin. It was horrendous. And not only that, the drugs are highly addictive. So of course, you can't just come off of them; you have to do one half pill at a time, usually, and it takes many months to do. Every six months you drop a little bit.

It took about eight years for me to come off all the drugs completely, with the switch to cannabis coming along with it. I transformed from using prescription drugs to using cannabis more and more frequently, trying more strains, with more edibles becoming available, and more CBD. You know, just more research was coming to light. So it took me quite some time to transfer over. And when I stopped all the prescription drugs, then it was time to start putting the weight on, and I used cannabis for that, too. Using raw cannabis, raw flower, raw leaves . . . making high density, high quality, basically plant-based protein shakes. So there's actually no high. Even though there's THC available, you don't heat it, you eat it, and that has a totally different effect on the body. But it still affected my appetite, and I started putting weight on, through the plant-based protein.

Now, I'm lifting weights and working out, as per the doctor, who is well-informed about cannabis, too. He was one of the top neurologists at the hospital until he recently left for the States. I've put on about sixty pounds in two and a half years, lifting weights and using plant-based protein, using hemp and cannabis together. There is no doubt that the hemp and cannabis have changed everything. And I'm also seizure-free. I haven't had a seizure in four years because of cannabis. I consider hemp and cannabis a superfood, absolutely, 100 percent. There's no doubt.

And I've been able to go back to work, too. They've been giving me a disability cheque for years, and I hate it. I hate every minute of it. So now this business has opened up—funny enough, a new cannabis company has come forward and asked me to run their micro grow. Now, the whole centre is ready, the whole building is ready, so we're pretty happy.

And while we're talking about the future, I'm interested to see where other therapies will go. Like [*the cannabinoid*] CBG. CBG gives a sense of relaxation but only from the neck down. There's no head high. So we're researching heavy CBG strains, because CBD and CBG together could be a very potent combination. I'm also really interested in the legalization of mushrooms. That's the next big thing in this country. We're detoxifying and applying to Health Canada for exemptions so that we can do small growing. We want to do a smaller study on epilepsy and magic mushrooms.

Advice to others? I'd say that if they're going to be using cannabis, start slow, be patient—patience you can't teach. Be patient with yourself, and in the end, you'll find the proper levels for you. Because every human body is different; everyone will react to THC and CBD differently. But when you find that sweet spot, it's life changing. I should know.

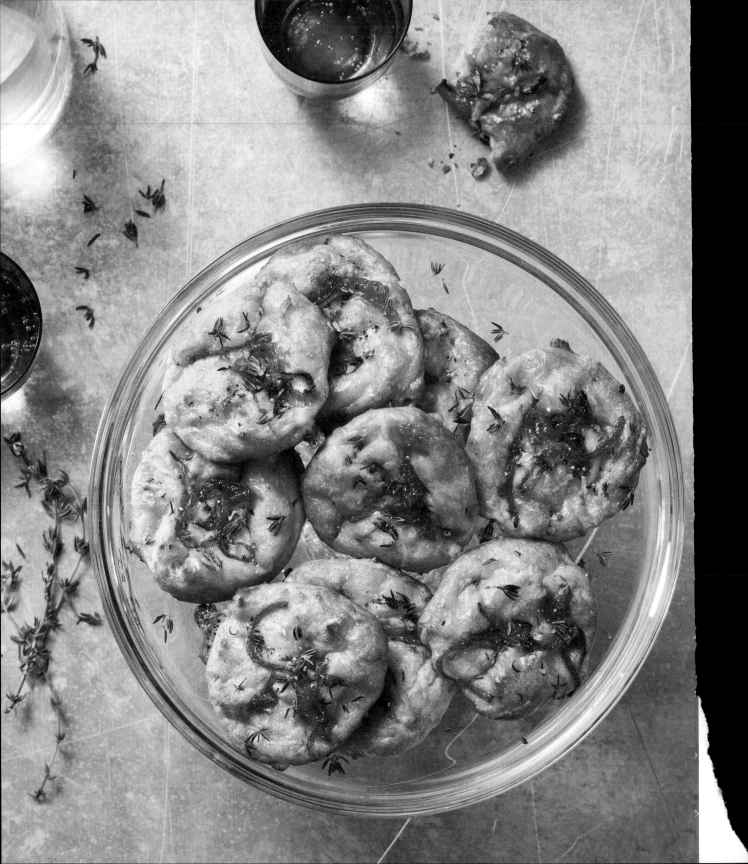

Caramelized Onion Blue Cheese Not-Gougères

Easier than explaining why blue cheese mould tastes good, these are "not-gougères" because the damn things wouldn't stay puffed for me. My food stylist extraordinaire, Carol, thought it was because the blue cheese was too heavy. But I wanted blue cheese! And they taste delicious. So I decided to go with their gentle lopsided deflations and invent something new. It really takes the stress out of life when you decide to give up on perfect and go with it.

SUGGESTED MOOD/STRAIN

Blue Cheese is an indica-dominant strain with relaxing, de-stressing effects.

Makes 40 cheese puffs with ½ cup cannabutter (almost 4 mg THC per piece).

¼ cup (57 g) unsalted butter
Glug of olive oil
2 large yellow onions, sliced into
    thin rounds
½ cup (113 g) cannabutter
½ cup (125 mL) milk (I used 1%)
1 cup (142 g) all-purpose flour
About 4 tsp fresh thyme, picked
    from the sprigs, divided
1 tsp cornstarch
A few dashes of salt
4 eggs, room temp
1 cup (227 g) blue cheese,
    crumbled
¼ cup (21 g) Parmesan cheese,
    grated

Start by caramelizing your onions. In a heavy pan, melt the regular butter with the olive oil. Add the onions and fry over medium heat, stirring occasionally, until they get deep brown—you'll notice the smell getting more decadent when they're close to done. Drain the liquids by pressing them out through a sieve over a bowl. (Fry something delicious for dinner in this fatty goodness.)

Preheat the oven to 400°F, and get your mixer and eggs ready. In a medium heavy-bottomed pot, melt the cannabutter. Add in the milk and a half cup of water, bringing it all to a boil. When it gets bubbly-crazy, reduce the heat to medium and add the cup of flour, stirring it with a wooden spoon until it comes together. In a small bowl, stir together half the thyme, ¼ cup of the onions (reserving at least 2 Tbsp or so for the topping), the cornstarch, and the salt, and add it to the dough. Keep turning the dough over with your wooden spoon, cooking it for about 3 minutes longer. You'll know it's ready when it starts making a mess of the bottom of your pot. (Leave that for your trusty non-cooking partner to scrub. I know I sure do.)

Dump the dough into your mixing bowl, and mix it a bit to help remove some of the heat. Add in the eggs, one at a time, incorporating each before adding the next, and being sure to scrape down the sides of the bowl a few times. Add the blue cheese.

Line a baking sheet with a silicone macaron mat.* Using two spoons, drop tall dollops onto the centres of the macaron circles. Don't overdo it here—they'll get a fair bit bigger after they bake. Try for about 1 Tbsp for each not-gougère. Top with the reserved thyme, reserved onions, and the Parmesan.

Bake for 15 minutes before reducing the oven temp to 350°F, without opening the oven door. Bake for an additional 5–10 minutes at the lower temperature until lovely and brown. You're welcome for the way your kitchen smells right now.

It's thyme for infused cheese puffs! (Sorry, couldn't resist.)

*A silicone macaron mat is helpful with sizing for this recipe, but not essential. You can also prep a baking sheet with a plain silicone mat or parchment paper, just be sure to space the puffs well and try to keep them evenly sized.

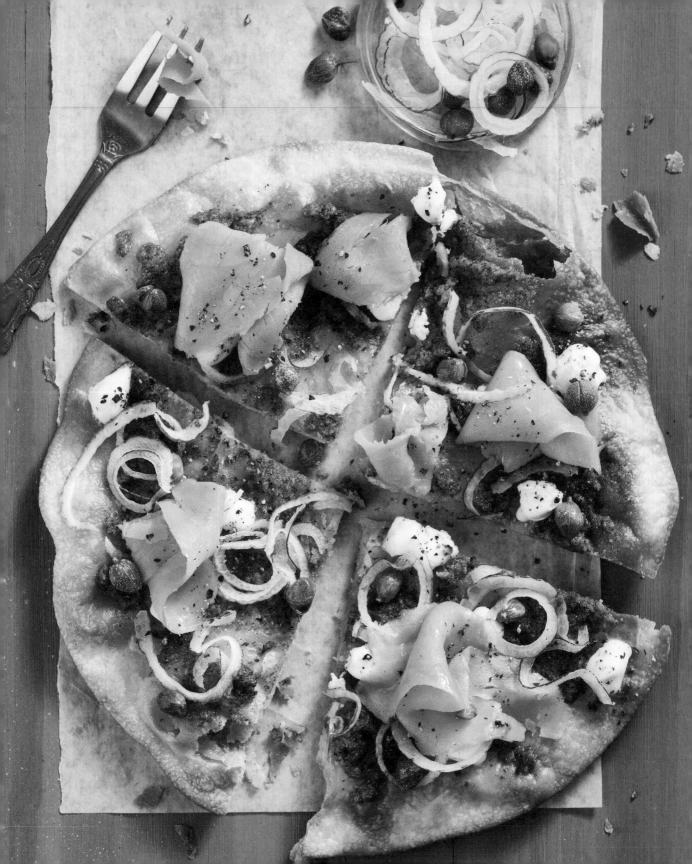

Smoked Salmon Goat Cheese Flatbreads with Pesto or Rosemary Garlic Sea-Salt Crackers

So here you have two appetizer options using the same basic components.
And both are easier than trying to come up with a never-before-seen pizza recipe.

SUGGESTED MOOD/STRAIN

Pizza Breath is a 50–50 hybrid that is said to smell like onions, mushrooms, and garlic.

The flatbread recipe makes 4 flatbreads cut into 4 pieces each, using ⅓ cup infused oil in total (about 4 mg THC per piece), which assumes 1 or 2 pieces per guest. If serving an entire flatbread to a guest, remember that 1 Tbsp of cannavirgin olive oil is about 11 mg THC, and adjust accordingly. The cracker recipe makes 60 crackers using ⅓ cup of infused olive oil (about 5 mg THC in 5 crackers).

Dough (Flatbreads or Crackers)

About 3 cups (414 g) 00 flour*
½ Tbsp sea salt + more salt if needed
⅓ cup (83 g) cannavirgin olive oil

Pesto Topping for Flatbreads

10 fresh basil leaves
¼ cup (27 g) pine nuts
2 garlic cloves
¼ cup (21 g) Parmesan, grated
Stream of extra-virgin olive oil

To make the dough for both the flatbreads and the crackers:
Using a mixer (I've even done this old school, with my hands), combine all dough ingredients, adding ¾ cups warm water very slowly at the end and stopping when the dough comes together. Divide the dough into quarters and knead each ball further. You're going for a smooth, soft, doughy (shocker) feel. If it's not coming together, add a bit more water, or just wet your hands and keep kneading. If it's too sticky, add a bit more flour.

On a smooth surface, roll each dough ball with a rolling pin onto a piece of parchment, as thin and flat as you can get it.

To make the flatbreads: Preheat oven to 450°F. Slide the dough rounds and parchment sheets directly onto the oven racks. Bake the crusts for about 8 minutes, but check them after 2 or 3 minutes for air bubbles. If the dough really puffed up (don't ask me how I know that it might), go ahead and pop the bubbles with a sharp knife. Remove each crust from the oven, flip it, slide it directly (upside down now) onto the oven rack, and bake for about 6 minutes more until the flatbreads are crisp and the edges are gently brown.

Meanwhile, make the pesto. (Honestly, please make it. I like to cheat as much as the next guy, but jarred pesto can be blech.) In a food processor, combine the basil, pine nuts, garlic, and Parmesan. Whizz it all together. Now, with the processor running, slowly pour a stream of olive oil in until the paste comes together and forms a sauce.

Preheat your oven broiler on high after the flatbreads come out of the oven. Spoon the pesto onto your doughs, smoothing it to all edges. Divide the goat cheese between the flatbreads in dollops. Sprinkle with red onion and capers. Broil the

**Goat Cheese and Smoked Salmon
  Topping for Flatbreads**

1 log (140 g) soft goat cheese

1-inch piece of red onion, sliced thin

4 Tbsp capers

Smoked salmon (140 g)

Rosemary Garlic Sea Salt Crackers

Extra-virgin olive oil

½ cup (42 g) freshly (finely) grated
  Parmesan

1 Tbsp fresh rosemary, chopped fine

1 Tbsp garlic powder

Sea salt to taste

flatbreads for about 2 or 3 minutes, making sure not to burn them.

Remove and decorate with pieces of smoked salmon. Slice with a pizza cutter and serve.

To make the crackers: Preheat oven to 450°F. Using the pizza cutter, slice off any uneven edges so that the dough shapes are perfect rectangles. Bring these cuttings together, roll out, and try for a few more crackers.

With a pastry brush, top the dough rectangles with olive oil. Sprinkle with Parmesan, rosemary, garlic powder, and sea salt. Using the pizza cutter again, slice the dough rectangles into squares.

Lift the parchment and one of the sliced dough pieces onto a baking sheet and slide it into the oven. Bake for about 8 minutes, flip the crackers with tongs, and bake about 6 minutes more, until crisp, but not browned. (Watch carefully.) Repeat with other dough pieces and bake crackers in batches.

These crackers actually get better if left in a bowl on the counter overnight, but no one will complain if they're served right away with cheese or dip (see page 205).

*You're going to have to find 00 flour. Hopefully, this isn't tricky where you live, but trust me, it's just so much better for pizzas/flatbreads—easier to work with because it rolls out so much thinner without the springiness, and also doesn't have that all-purpose taste.

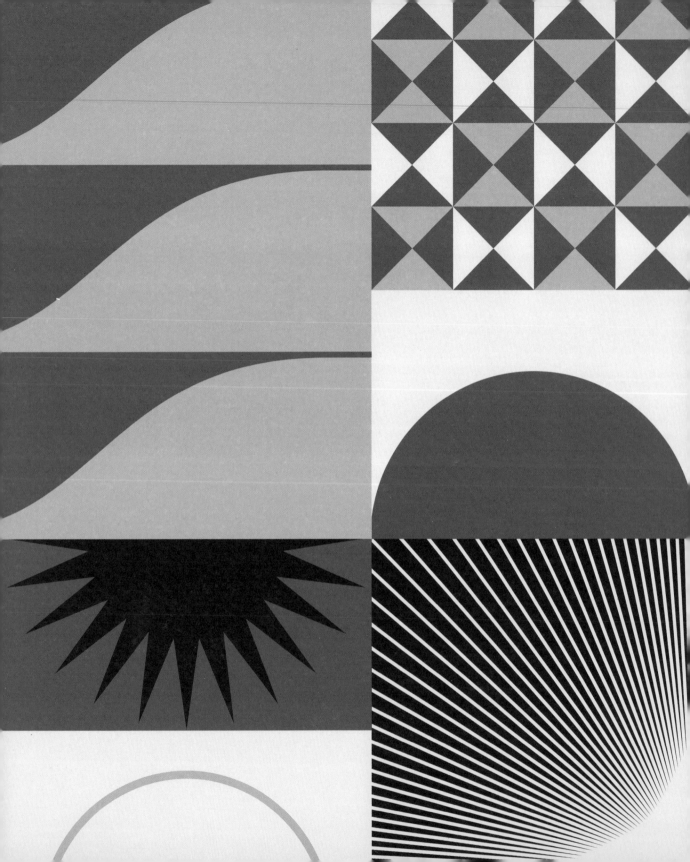

THE
GREAT
PEACH
GUMMY

RECIPE

STORY

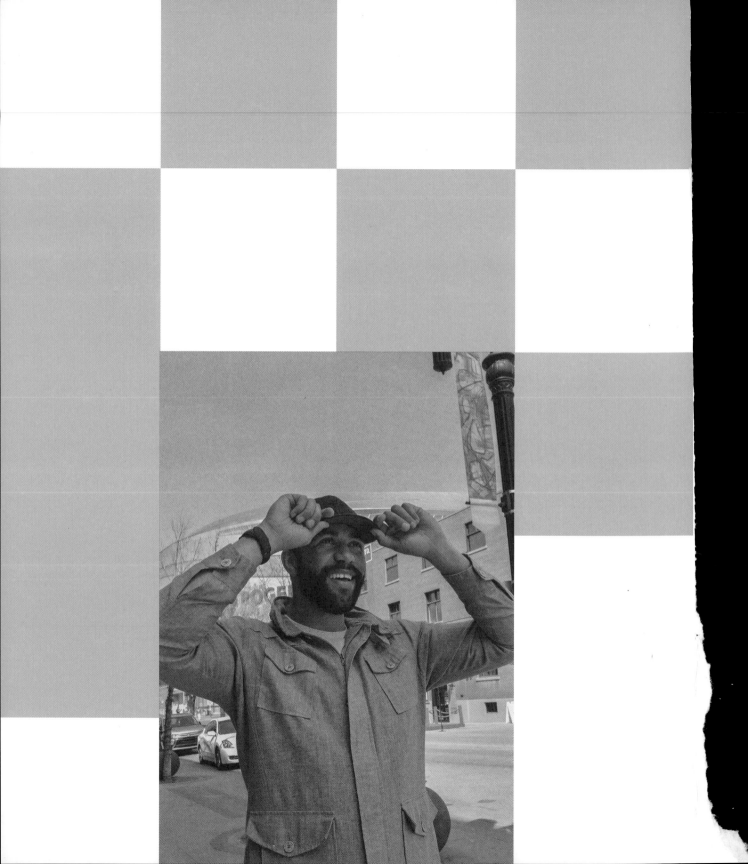

Keenan Pascal

Keenan Pascal is CEO of Token Naturals, a cannabis processor and product development company based in Edmonton, Alberta. Keenan also formed the Black Canadians Cannabis Network, a networking organization for cannabis professionals.

As a youth, I wasn't really big into cannabis but my interest was sparked around 2014. I was doing my MBA at UBC [*University of British Columbia*], and one of my classmates had worked in the grey market as a grower and was very in tune with the plant. He made drinks and cocktails for us, subbing out alcohol and adding cannabis in its place. We started talking about the benefits of consumption from a health standpoint, and I was definitely intrigued, because you know, as you get older, hangovers get uglier, and I was very health-focused in terms of fitness. With cannabis, I'd have a night out in Vancouver and wake up in the morning and still be able to go on a hike. Later, I explored more with CBD, and now I take CBD every morning as part of my health and fitness routine. It's just something I really enjoy as a recovery tool and as an alternative to liquor.

But the real excitement for me in the cannabis space was when we started our company, Token Naturals. When we launched Token in 2016, we knew we had a long regulatory process ahead of us and a lot of waiting time for licensing. To put that time to good use, we started a small cocktail bitters company—Token

Bitters—to learn more about extraction and product development. We grew it from my garage to become the biggest bitters company in Alberta, then expanded to selling across Canada and even to Japan. That bitters company is still going, but now that we have our cannabis licence, we're making cannabis products, too. In cannabis, we're making our own Token-branded products, and we're creating products for businesses. One group of clients is licensed producers that want to turn their flower into processed products, such as oils or topicals, because they don't have the capacity, space, or equipment in-house to do so. What really excites me are the up-and-coming brands that approach us to make their products. Those are the people who have a really interesting non-cannabis product that they want to infuse with cannabis. They might be chefs or athletes who want to put CBD in their favourite salve, or someone who is bringing a unique beverage recipe into Canada and adding THC to it. Those conversations are what really excite us now, the new brands. We've only seen the tip of the iceberg in terms of innovation and what the range of products is going to look like.

We built out this cannabis manufacturing facility, and that's when we started to get a lot of attention for being a very diverse business. We're a Black-led company, and our investor pool is 70 percent people of colour and/or female. And there was such opportunity coming into this new cannabis industry to hire a diverse team. If you're thinking about an engineer, you might think you know what that person is going to look like when they walk into the room. But with cannabis, you can go to a bunch of different meetings and—especially in the early stages—you are meeting such a range of people with different backgrounds and experiences. Because of the capital requirements needed to begin operating in this regulatory framework, there was the concern that the diversity was getting erased. But that's been critically noticed, and I see changes already in terms of regulation, task forces, and structural support. Diversity is at the forefront of everybody's mind in the cannabis space; it's not something that's just being sidelined, which is refreshing.

Then the Black Lives Matter movement drew mass attention with the murder of George Floyd, and there was a big flood of people asking, "Hey, where are the Black people in Canadian cannabis?"

I'm lucky enough to be well-networked in the space, so a lot of people turned and asked me, and I myself didn't even know. So, I put out a LinkedIn post with that question. That led to the creation of our group, the Black Canadians Cannabis Network, which now has about seventy members, and we've been growing steadily. The network is fairly informal; we'll jump on a call together and discuss pain points and upcoming opportunities. It's like, "Oh, you need someone in marketing? Talk to Kyle, or Zola, or Evan. If you need manufacturing, talk to Keenan. If you need a grower, here's Nathan." You're seeing these conversations starting to work together, which I think is probably the most interesting part that's come up so far. As we grow, we'll add more mentorship to it and projects with Health Canada to get more inclusion and involvement.

The future for Token? We're going to continue to build out manufacturing capacity for the industry. Edmonton's been a great city to set up shop. It's so wide open with opportunity. You can pick up the phone

if you want to talk to somebody that's one or two degrees of separation away and get an introduction. It's a big city, small-town vibe. We've built out our manufacturing facility here in microblocks, and that was a different take, because everyone was always rushing to just jump in and be the first, and the fastest, and the biggest, but we thought: let's take this one step at a time and prove our concept responsibly. That strategy has paid off as we've been scaling up slowly and steadily. Now, we're working hard to show that Edmonton holds the best opportunities for cannabis processing.

We're really excited to bring some cool brands to the market, especially ours. We're starting in the drink additive space with a brand called Favour, a THC or CBD "shot" that you can take straight or make a mocktail with. Seeing people start getting creative, make new cool products, bring in new genetics, and reduce the stigmatization of the plant is what I'm looking forward to most in the future. I want to see more of those social experiences where you bring over a six-pack of cannabis drinks and nobody looks at you funny. Cannabis is increasingly out in the open, rather than needing to be discrete. An exciting experience for me has been having friends over, maybe watching a game, and most of us are trying a gummy or sipping on a cannabis beverage instead of just pounding back beer after beer.

We're all about building community at Token. So, we're focused on collaboration throughout the industry and reducing barriers to entry as much as possible. We want to advance the industry as a whole to set up a scenario where, when we win, so do our partners, so does Edmonton, and so does the industry at large.

Peach Gummies

Easier than really loving peaches and shaking someone's tree.
I wanted the perfect gummy recipe and I got one! From Alina
(although dosing and shape are my own). Alina makes infused candies
on her YouTube channel, *Alina's Best Buds*. She's super cute and talented
with her infusions, so please go follow her.

SUGGESTED MOOD/STRAIN

Peach OG is an indica-dominant hybrid that gives a fairly light buzz.

Makes 24 1½-inch gummies with 15 mL tincture concentrate (almost 4 mg THC per piece).

Potassium Sorbate Solution

1 Tbsp potassium sorbate

3 Tbsp water

Tincture Reduction

10½ g decarboxylated cannabis flower* (¼ oz + ⅛ oz)

½ cup (120 mL) highest proof alcohol available

Gummies

3½ Tbsp gelatin

1 tsp citric acid

1 tsp concentrated peach flavouring; ¼ tsp if it's the "4 times as strong" stuff

1½ tsp lecithin

¼ cup (50 g) granulated sugar

¼ cup (63 mL) corn syrup

Gathering your supplies: I'll admit this recipe calls for some rather niche pantry supplies! Potassium sorbate helps with gummy shelf life. Order through that online retailer we love to hate. Slight cash outlay, but the amount will last a lifetime. Citric acid and lecithin (mine was soy) can be found at bulk stores or online. Concentrated peach flavouring can be ordered online or from a cake supplies retailer. The cannabis leaf silicone candy moulds: Mine came in a set of 3 for a total of 24 gummies—the perfect amount for this recipe. You can use any candy silicone moulds, but I prefer the cannabis type so that it's obvious that the gummies are infused.

To make the potassium sorbate solution: Combine potassium sorbate with water. Store excess in a wee jar—you'll only need ¼ tsp right now.

To make the tincture reduction: In another (jam-sized) jar, combine decarboxylated cannabis with enough alcohol to cover it. Let it sit on the counter and infuse for at least 45 minutes, preferably longer, shaking it here and there. Sieve the weed out through a cheesecloth, wringing out as much liquid as possible.

Now let's boil off some of the alcohol. In a small pot on the stove, heat the alcohol over low heat until it gets down to less than ¼ cup, about 15 minutes. But take care. Don't ask how I know this, but alcohol on a stove can be flammable. Keep a pot lid nearby and do NOT leave your concoction alone. If it should happen to flame, keep calm, whisper "Opa," to yourself, shut the heat off, and cover it with a pot lid.

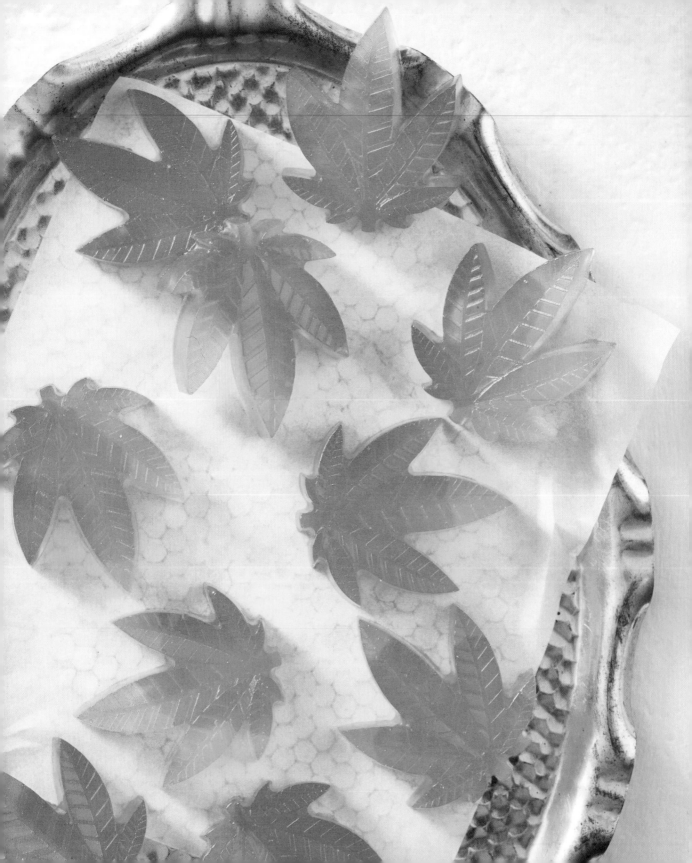

Notes

1. Drug Policy Alliance. "Debunking the 'Gateway' Myth." (February 2017): drugpolicy.org/sites/default/files/DebunkingGatewayMyth_NY_0.pdf

2. Lachenmeier, Rehm. "Comparative Risk Assessment of Alcohol, Tobacco, Cannabis and Other Illicit Drugs Using the Margin of Exposure Approach." *Sci Rep* (2015): 8126.

Ben-Shabat, Fride, Sheskin, Tamiri, Rhee, Vogel, et al. "An Entourage Effect: active Endogenous Fatty Acid Glycerol Esters Enhance 2-Arachidonoyl-Glycerol annabinoid Activity." *European Journal of Pharmacology* 353, no.1 (July 1998): 8–31.

Pellati, Federica, Borgonetti, Vittoria, Brighenti, Virginia, et al. "*Cannabis tiva* L. and Non-Psychoactive Cannabinoids: Their Chemistry and Role Against idative Stress, Inflammation, and Cancer." *BioMed Research International*. (2018): .org/10.1155/2018/1691428.

Tramèr, Martin, Carroll, Dawn, Campbell, Fiona, et al. "Cannabinoids for ntrol of Chemotherapy Induced Nausea and Vomiting: Quantitative Systematic iew." *The BMJ* 323 (2001): 16.

lake, Alexia, Wan, Bo Angela, Malek, Leila, et al. "A Selective Review of Medical nabis in Cancer Pain Management." *Annals of Palliative Medicine* 6, Supplement ugust 23, 2017): S215–S222.

otz, Janine, Fehlmann, Bernhard, Papassortiropoulos, Andreas, et al. nabidiol Enhances Verbal Episodic Memory in Healthy Young Participants: A lomized Clinical Trial." *Journal of Psychiatric Research* 143 (2021): 327–333.

ate, Giulia, Uberti, Daniela, Tambaro, Simone. "Potential and Limits of abinoids in Alzheimer's Disease Therapy." Biology 10, no. 6 (June 2021): 542; i, Federica, Borgonetti, Vittoria, Brighenti, Virginia, et al. "Cannabis Sativa L. Non-Psychoactive Cannabinoids: Their Chemistry and Role Against Oxidative

To make the gummies: Bloom your gelatin by sprinkling it over ⅓ cup of water. Continue the sprinklage (enjoying that word?) with ¼ tsp potassium sorbate solution, the citric acid, the peach flavouring, and the lecithin, without stirring. Let this sit for at least 5 minutes.

In a small saucepan, heat the sugar with the corn syrup over medium-high heat until the sugar melts and it gets bubbly. Clip on the candy thermometer. Boil water in the kettle, and have two small dishes that will fit into a larger basin nearby (a big pie plate or rimmed baking pan), in prep for a water bath.

Add half of the gelatin mixture to the sugar and corn syrup and whisk until it melts. Heat to between 200°F and 210°F (this happens quickly, so keep an eye out), remove from heat, and add in the remaining gelatin mixture. Whisk in the tincture reduction.

Pour the not-yet-gummy liquid into the two small dishes and place them into the larger basin/pan/dish. Fill the basin with boiling water from the kettle, letting it come midway up the dishes. This will keep the gummy liquid warm in its wee bath. Colour one dish yellow and the other orange with the gel food colourings.

Pour the yellow not-yet-gummy liquid through the funnel and into one of the squeeze bottles. Squeeze little bits into some of the leaf moulds, leaving halves of them empty, ready for some orange. Don't use it all up. Put the yellow squeeze bottle directly into the water bath (keeping it warm), and fill the other squeeze bottle with orange. Add orange and yellow interchangeably to the moulds until all 24 are full.

Freeze the moulds for 30 minutes. Deep breath. The gummies should be good to go! Go ahead and turn them out of the moulds, and peach it up.

*See page 27 for directions on how to decarboxylate cannabis. I sent the first batch of gummies I made to the lab, and the dosing sucked. So here, you're going to purchase higher THC cannabis than what I recommend for butter—let's try for between 25 and 30 percent.

Acknowledgem

Well, isn't it just like me that this is the very last part of the
The most important part. I guess it's a bit like an Oscars spe
you forget someone while the clock is ticking, it was for th
your husband).

So, let's start with my husband. Phil has been here ever
behind me, cleaning up hundreds of dishes. He was the fir
edibles—he popped two cookies before I knew what I wa
for a run, came back, and struggled to talk. He's also my

Thanks to the rest of my family, too, including Charly
and Frank, John and Janet, my aunts and uncles, my cou
My family is so warm that it's almost dysfunctional; havi
was nerve-wracking but they took it in stride. I knew th
was doing, I didn't care what anyone else thought.

Thanks to Kishma, Mel (even Bryan), the slummy r
friends. Thanks to my early secret dealers (you know w
the-alley horticulturalist friend, Chris. Thanks to Hon
helped me with ideas and slip-ups all the way through

Full pause (that sounded lame, but this needs to b
written this without the stories, and the openness of e
about their cannabis histories. I'm so glad that all of y
well-being through this plant, and that you've encou
your honesty. Alan, Sarah, Reena, and Andi, you fou
Chris and Aud, you went to prison for what I'm end
sugar. I'm glad you made it through. Thank you.

Amana/Ari and Highness Global, you gave this
TouchWood. Thank you for believing in the potent
only exists because of the creativity and vision of C
quarterback, and baking coach; Christine Hanlon,
Jodi Pudge, the world-class (and endlessly pleasan

Lastly, thanks to Kathie (and my father-in-law
me, sharing your story when you've seen many m
even one person tries cannabis medicinally becau
it's you they have to thank.

Stress, Inflammation, and Cancer." *BioMed Research International*. (2018): doi. org/10.1155/2018/1691428.

9. Zaheer, Sidra, Kumar, Deepak, Khan, Muhammed T., et al. "Epilepsy and Cannabis: A Literature Review." *Cureus* 10, no. 9 (September 2018): e3278.

10. Namdar, Dvory, Koltai, Hinait. "Medical Cannabis for the Treatment of Inflammation." *National Product Communications* 13, no. 13 (2018): 249–254.

11. Russo, Ethan. "Cannabis Treatments in Obstetrics and Gynecology: A Historical Review." *Journal of Cannabis Therapeutics* 2 Issue 3–4 (2002): 5–35.

12. Cuttler, Carrie, Spradlin, Alexander, Cleveland, Michael J., et al. "Short- and Long-Term Effects of Cannabis on Headache and Migraine." *The Journal of Pain* 21, no. 5–6 (May/June 2020): 722–730.

13. Ige, Maryam, Liu, Ji. "Herbal Medicines in Glaucoma Treatment." *Yale Journal of Biology and Medicine* 93, no. 2 (June 2020): 347–353.

14. Lucas, Phillipe, Walsh, Zach, Crosby, Kim, et al. "Substituting Cannabis for Prescription Drugs, Alcohol and Other Substances Among Medical Cannabis Patients: The Impact of Contextual Factors." *Drug and Alcohol Review* 35 (2016): 326–333.

15. Risso, Constanza, Boniface, Sadie, Subbaraman, Meenaskhi Sabina, et al. "Does Cannabis Complement or Substitute Alcohol Consumption? A Systematic Review of Human and Animal Studies." *Journal of Psychopharmacology* 34, no 3 (2020): 938–954.

16. Blevins, Dumic. "The Effect of Delta-9-Tetrahydrocannabinol on Herpes Simplex Virus Replication." *J Gen Virol* 49(2) (August 1980): 427–31.

17. Volkow, Nora, Baler, Ruben, Compton, Wilson, et al. "Adverse Health Effects of Marijuana Use." *New England Journal of Medicine* 370 (2014): 2219–2227.

18. Zehra, Amna, Burns, Jamie, Lu, Christopher Kure, et al. "Cannabis Addiction and the Brain: a Review." *Journal of Neuroimmune Pharmacology* 13, no. 4 (2018): 438–452.

19. Karila, Laurent, Roux, Perrine, Rolland, Benjamin, et al. "Acute and Long-Term Effects of Cannabis Use: A Review." *Current Pharmaceutical Design* 20 (2014): 4112–4118; Katz, Gregory, Lobel, Tsafrir, Tetelbaum, Alex, et al. "Cannabis Withdrawal—A New Diagnostic Category in DSM-5." *The Israel Journal of Psychiatry and Related Sciences* 51 (2014): 270–275.

20. Colizzi, Marco, Bhattacharyya, Sagnik. "Cannabis Use and the Development of Tolerance: A Systematic Review of Human Evidence." *Neuroscience & Biobehavioral Reviews* 93 (October 2018): 1–25.

21. Rodrigo, Chaturaka, Rajapakse, Senaka. "Cannabis and Schizophrenia Spectrum Disorders: A Review of Clinical Studies." *Indian Journal of Psychological Medicine* 31, no. 2 (July–December 2009): 62–70.

22. There is some debate about formal cannabis taxonomy, but I'm going with *Cannabis* for the genus win, as recommended by Pollio, in "The name of *Cannabis*: A short guide for Nonbotanists," https://www.ncbi.nlm.nih.gov/pmc/articles/PMC5531363/. 2016; 1(1): 234–238.

Stress, Inflammation, and Cancer." *BioMed Research International*. (2018): doi. org/10.1155/2018/1691428.

9. Zaheer, Sidra, Kumar, Deepak, Khan, Muhammed T., et al. "Epilepsy and Cannabis: A Literature Review." *Cureus* 10, no. 9 (September 2018): e3278.

10. Namdar, Dvory, Koltai, Hinait. "Medical Cannabis for the Treatment of Inflammation." *National Product Communications* 13, no. 13 (2018): 249–254.

11. Russo, Ethan. "Cannabis Treatments in Obstetrics and Gynecology: A Historical Review." *Journal of Cannabis Therapeutics* 2 Issue 3–4 (2002): 5–35.

12. Cuttler, Carrie, Spradlin, Alexander, Cleveland, Michael J., et al. "Short- and Long-Term Effects of Cannabis on Headache and Migraine." *The Journal of Pain* 21, no. 5–6 (May/June 2020): 722–730.

13. Ige, Maryam, Liu, Ji. "Herbal Medicines in Glaucoma Treatment." *Yale Journal of Biology and Medicine* 93, no. 2 (June 2020): 347–353.

14. Lucas, Phillipe, Walsh, Zach, Crosby, Kim, et al. "Substituting Cannabis for Prescription Drugs, Alcohol and Other Substances Among Medical Cannabis Patients: The Impact of Contextual Factors." *Drug and Alcohol Review* 35 (2016): 326–333.

15. Risso, Constanza, Boniface, Sadie, Subbaraman, Meenaskhi Sabina, et al. "Does Cannabis Complement or Substitute Alcohol Consumption? A Systematic Review of Human and Animal Studies." *Journal of Psychopharmacology* 34, no 3 (2020): 938–954.

16. Blevins, Dumic. "The Effect of Delta-9-Tetrahydrocannabinol on Herpes Simplex Virus Replication." *J Gen Virol* 49(2) (August 1980): 427–31.

17. Volkow, Nora, Baler, Ruben, Compton, Wilson, et al. "Adverse Health Effects of Marijuana Use." *New England Journal of Medicine* 370 (2014): 2219–2227.

18. Zehra, Amna, Burns, Jamie, Lu, Christopher Kure, et al. "Cannabis Addiction and the Brain: a Review." *Journal of Neuroimmune Pharmacology* 13, no. 4 (2018): 438–452.

19. Karila, Laurent, Roux, Perrine, Rolland, Benjamin, et al. "Acute and Long-Term Effects of Cannabis Use: A Review." *Current Pharmaceutical Design* 20 (2014): 4112–4118; Katz, Gregory, Lobel, Tsafrir, Tetelbaum, Alex, et al. "Cannabis Withdrawal—A New Diagnostic Category in DSM-5." *The Israel Journal of Psychiatry and Related Sciences* 51 (2014): 270–275.

20. Colizzi, Marco, Bhattacharyya, Sagnik. "Cannabis Use and the Development of Tolerance: A Systematic Review of Human Evidence." *Neuroscience & Biobehavioral Reviews* 93 (October 2018): 1–25.

21. Rodrigo, Chaturaka, Rajapakse, Senaka. "Cannabis and Schizophrenia Spectrum Disorders: A Review of Clinical Studies." *Indian Journal of Psychological Medicine* 31, no. 2 (July–December 2009): 62–70.

22. There is some debate about formal cannabis taxonomy, but I'm going with *Cannabis* for the genus win, as recommended by Pollio, in "The name of *Cannabis*: A short guide for Nonbotanists," https://www.ncbi.nlm.nih.gov/pmc/articles/PMC5531363/. 2016; 1(1): 234–238.

To make the gummies: Bloom your gelatin by sprinkling it over ⅓ cup of water. Continue the sprinklage (enjoying that word?) with ¼ tsp potassium sorbate solution, the citric acid, the peach flavouring, and the lecithin, without stirring. Let this sit for at least 5 minutes.

In a small saucepan, heat the sugar with the corn syrup over medium-high heat until the sugar melts and it gets bubbly. Clip on the candy thermometer. Boil water in the kettle, and have two small dishes that will fit into a larger basin nearby (a big pie plate or rimmed baking pan), in prep for a water bath.

Add half of the gelatin mixture to the sugar and corn syrup and whisk until it melts. Heat to between 200°F and 210°F (this happens quickly, so keep an eye out), remove from heat, and add in the remaining gelatin mixture. Whisk in the tincture reduction.

Pour the not-yet-gummy liquid into the two small dishes and place them into the larger basin/pan/dish. Fill the basin with boiling water from the kettle, letting it come midway up the dishes. This will keep the gummy liquid warm in its wee bath. Colour one dish yellow and the other orange with the gel food colourings.

Pour the yellow not-yet-gummy liquid through the funnel and into one of the squeeze bottles. Squeeze little bits into some of the leaf moulds, leaving halves of them empty, ready for some orange. Don't use it all up. Put the yellow squeeze bottle directly into the water bath (keeping it warm), and fill the other squeeze bottle with orange. Add orange and yellow interchangeably to the moulds until all 24 are full.

Freeze the moulds for 30 minutes. Deep breath. The gummies should be good to go! Go ahead and turn them out of the moulds, and peach it up.

*See page 27 for directions on how to decarboxylate cannabis. I sent the first batch of gummies I made to the lab, and the dosing sucked. So here, you're going to purchase higher THC cannabis than what I recommend for butter—let's try for between 25 and 30 percent.

Acknowledgements

Well, isn't it just like me that this is the very last part of the manuscript I'm finishing? The most important part. I guess it's a bit like an Oscars speech, though, where if you forget someone while the clock is ticking, it was for the best anyway (unless it's your husband).

So, let's start with my husband. Phil has been here every step of the way, literally behind me, cleaning up hundreds of dishes. He was the first person ever to try my edibles—he popped two cookies before I knew what I was doing with dosing, went for a run, came back, and struggled to talk. He's also my greatest cheerleader.

Thanks to the rest of my family, too, including Charly and Reid, my parents, Jen and Frank, John and Janet, my aunts and uncles, my cousins, and the Irish cousins. My family is so warm that it's almost dysfunctional; having them embrace this book was nerve-wracking but they took it in stride. I knew that if they accepted what I was doing, I didn't care what anyone else thought.

Thanks to Kishma, Mel (even Bryan), the slummy mummies, and my other dear friends. Thanks to my early secret dealers (you know who you are), and to my across-the-alley horticulturalist friend, Chris. Thanks to Hong, my baking mentor, who has helped me with ideas and slip-ups all the way through this journey.

Full pause (that sounded lame, but this needs to be set apart)—I couldn't have written this without the stories, and the openness of everyone who spoke with me about their cannabis histories. I'm so glad that all of you have found health and well-being through this plant, and that you've encouraged others to do the same with your honesty. Alan, Sarah, Reena, and Andi, you fought the law, and the weed won. Chris and Aud, you went to prison for what I'm endlessly mixing into butter and sugar. I'm glad you made it through. Thank you.

Amana/Ari and Highness Global, you gave this book life. So did you, TouchWood. Thank you for believing in the potential. And the beauty of the book only exists because of the creativity and vision of Carol Dudar, the food stager, quarterback, and baking coach; Christine Hanlon, props stager extraordinaire; and Jodi Pudge, the world-class (and endlessly pleasant and patient) food photographer.

Lastly, thanks to Kathie (and my father-in-law John). You've been so open with me, sharing your story when you've seen many more years of stigma than I have. If even one person tries cannabis medicinally because they're welcomed by this book, it's you they have to thank.

Notes

1. Drug Policy Alliance. "Debunking the 'Gateway' Myth." (February 2017): drugpolicy.org/sites/default/files/DebunkingGatewayMyth_NY_0.pdf

2. Lachenmeier, Rehm. "Comparative Risk Assessment of Alcohol, Tobacco, Cannabis and Other Illicit Drugs Using the Margin of Exposure Approach." *Sci Rep* 5 (2015): 8126.

3. Ben-Shabat, Fride, Sheskin, Tamiri, Rhee, Vogel, et al. "An Entourage Effect: Inactive Endogenous Fatty Acid Glycerol Esters Enhance 2-Arachidonoyl-Glycerol Cannabinoid Activity." *European Journal of Pharmacology* 353, no.1 (July 1998): 23–31.

4. Pellati, Federica, Borgonetti, Vittoria, Brighenti, Virginia, et al. "*Cannabis Sativa* L. and Non-Psychoactive Cannabinoids: Their Chemistry and Role Against Oxidative Stress, Inflammation, and Cancer." *BioMed Research International*. (2018): doi.org/10.1155/2018/1691428.

5. Tramèr, Martin, Carroll, Dawn, Campbell, Fiona, et al. "Cannabinoids for Control of Chemotherapy Induced Nausea and Vomiting: Quantitative Systematic Review." *The BMJ* 323 (2001): 16.

6. Blake, Alexia, Wan, Bo Angela, Malek, Leila, et al. "A Selective Review of Medical Cannabis in Cancer Pain Management." *Annals of Palliative Medicine* 6, Supplement 2 (August 23, 2017): S215–S222.

7. Hotz, Janine, Fehlmann, Bernhard, Papassortiropoulos, Andreas, et al. "Cannabidiol Enhances Verbal Episodic Memory in Healthy Young Participants: A Randomized Clinical Trial." *Journal of Psychiatric Research* 143 (2021): 327–333.

8. Abate, Giulia, Uberti, Daniela, Tambaro, Simone. "Potential and Limits of Cannabinoids in Alzheimer's Disease Therapy." Biology 10, no. 6 (June 2021): 542; Pellati, Federica, Borgonetti, Vittoria, Brighenti, Virginia, et al. "Cannabis Sativa L. and Non-Psychoactive Cannabinoids: Their Chemistry and Role Against Oxidative

Index

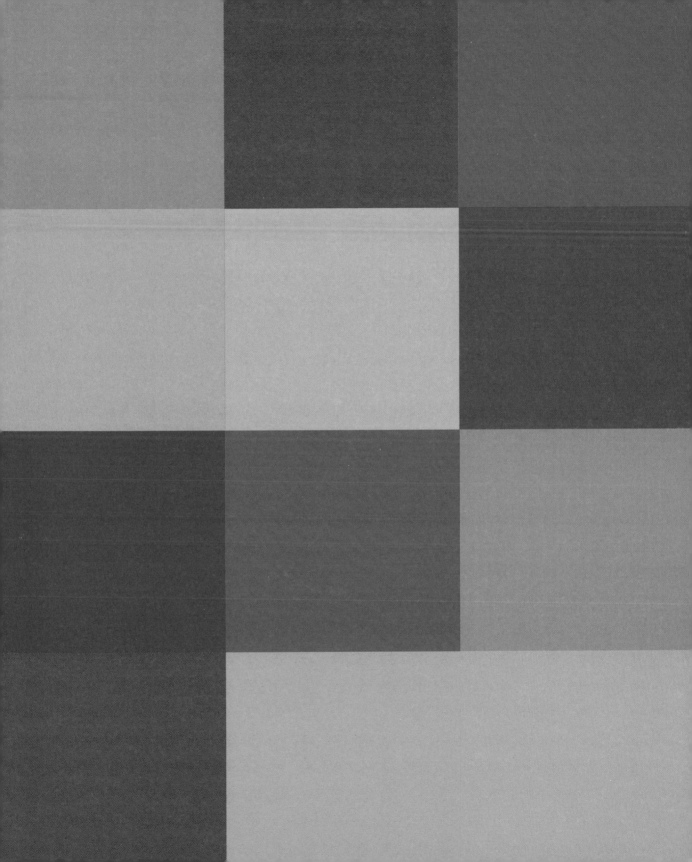

TouchWood Editions
touchwoodeditions.com

Interior photos by Jodi Pudge
Food staging by Carol Dudar
Props staging by Christine Hanlon
Photos accompanying the stories appear courtesy of the interviewees
Cover and interior design by Tree Abraham
Edited by Paula Marchese

Cataloguing information available from Library and Archives Canada
ISBN 9781771513708 (hardcover)
ISBN 9781771513715 (electronic)

TouchWood Editions acknowledges that the land on which we live and work is within
the traditional territories of the Lkwungen (Esquimalt and Songhees), Malahat, Pacheedaht,
Scia'new, T'sou-ke and W̱SÁNEĆ (Pauquachin, Tsartlip, Tsawout, Tseycum) peoples.

We acknowledge the financial support of the Government of Canada through the Canada
Book Fund, and the Province of British Columbia through the Book Publishing Tax Credit.

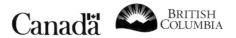

This book was printed using FSC-certified, acid-free papers, processed chlorine free,
and printed with soya-based inks.

Printed in China

26 25 24 23 22   1 2 3 4 5